THE Microbiology Bench Companion

THE Microbiology Bench Companion

J. Michael Miller, Ph.D., (D)ABMM
Microbiology Technical Services
Dunwoody, Georgia

ASM PRESS **Washington, DC**

Address editorial correspondence to ASM Press, 1752 N St. NW,
Washington, DC 20036-2904, USA

Send orders to ASM Press, P.O. Box 605, Herndon, VA 20172, USA
Phone: (800) 546-2416 or (703) 661-1593
Fax: (703) 661-1501
E-mail: books@asmusa.org
Online: estore.asm.org

Library of Congress Cataloging-in-Publication Data

Miller, J. Michael (Jon Michael), 1945–
The microbiology bench companion / J. Michael Miller.
p. cm.
Includes bibliographical references and index.
ISBN-13: 978-1-55581-402-1 (pbk.)
1. Medical microbiology—Handbooks, manuals, etc. I. Title.

QR46.M585 2007
616.9′041—dc22

2007060371

10 9 8 7 6 5 4 3 2 1

Contents

Preface

As clinical microbiologists and for clients of the microbiology laboratory, we have been privileged to have a plethora of wonderful texts and manuals, written by the bright leaders in the field, that make our role on the health care team a viable contribution to excellent patient care. Assisting in the diagnosis of infectious diseases has a considerable impact on patient outcome, infection control, and the cost of patient care, and it provides a significant degree of comfort to clinicians charged with diagnosis and therapeutic response.

Microbiology is becoming more complex, not simpler, because of the living organisms we interact with daily. Like moving targets, any of these microorganisms that we detect or culture may or may not be the etiologic agent responsible for specific symptoms. They may or may not be susceptible to the antimicrobics empirically prescribed by attending physicians. They may or may not be easily cultivatable in the laboratory or even easily coaxed from the specimen submitted for analysis. In fact, they may or may not be part of the normal flora in an individual. Optimizing the contributions of the microbiology laboratory requires an expertise not usually exhibited by generalists who are required to rotate through microbiology during the course of their work schedules. Clinical microbiology is a science of interpretive judgment requiring extensive specialty training in order to provide clinicians the complete information they need.

Ideally, every clinical microbiology laboratory should be directed by a specialist certified by the American Board of Medical Microbiology or the American Board of Medical Laboratory Immunology or their equivalents, or it should have direct access to such board-certified specialists. Hiring and retaining certified microbiology specialists in this complex field should be just as attractive and necessary to hospital chief executive officers and laboratory medical directors as employing board-certified clinicians and surgeons is, since certification is clearly documentation of expertise and quality.

This book is written primarily for those microbiology laboratorians who do not have access to these experts. I have immense respect for those individuals who work at the bench in the clinical microbiology laboratory. They tend to be astute, highly capable professionals who are asked difficult questions on a daily basis, and my sense is that they would always love to have a little more information at their fingertips to fully satisfy a questioning physician or even a laboratory colleague. Many texts are available to provide specific identification techniques and even photographs of isolates, but few of these books offer convenient caveats that are directly related to the organism(s) isolated and reported and that help "decode" what is going on.

The Microbiology Bench Companion is an easy reference to be used by the technologist, nurse, or physician to assist in "decoding" an organism that has just been reported. I realize that many experienced microbiologists and our board-certified colleagues probably know every piece of information presented in these tables and charts, but this book will serve as a handy reference for them too. More importantly, virtually everything I have learned in microbiology was learned from someone else without whose expertise I would still be struggling more than I am. For that, I am eternally grateful to a myriad of colleagues who continue to amaze me with their knowledge and their willingness to share it. I would never overlook an opportunity to acknowledge a source of information, but in this work I have surely omitted some originators of a piece of advice or an astute observation made in the last 30 years, and for that I apologize. In addition, with the advent of genomics, so easily and effectively applied to taxonomy, it is clear that nomenclature changes, additions, and deletions occur seemingly with each journal publication. I recommend that as those changes occur, the reader simply make a marginal note in the text and hope that the next edition of the *Companion* will include the new or modified names.

The idea for the format of the information in this book actually came from my colleague and friend Harvey H. Holmes, who used a similar approach for his laboratorians when he directed a microbiology laboratory at a large medical center. Building on his idea, the *Companion* stands ready to offer small but significant bits of information about the most common organisms we see in the clinical microbiology arena.

SECTION I
Decisions at the Bench

How To Use *The Microbiology Bench Companion*

The Microbiology Bench Companion is designed to serve as a guide for the technologist working at the laboratory bench when a question arises about a specific organism regarding

1. Unique identifying features
2. Determining whether a susceptibility test can be done
3. Providing published information about drugs of choice
4. Classifying difficult organisms by using a few simple tests

The *Companion* is divided into three main sections.

Section I consists of a table suggesting the level of accuracy expected for a report from an automated system followed by a group of 13 algorithms for placing unknown isolates into general groups for further workup. The algorithm lines are interpreted as follows: arrows to the right mean "yes or positive," and arrows downward mean "no or negative."

Section II contains some minimal susceptibility testing parameters and the limits of such testing. Also included are some bench observations that should be familiar to technologists who routinely work up organisms and note some specific, unusual, or special features of certain isolates. In addition, a table that associates the possible and expected isolates from some of the more commonly discussed infectious diseases is included.

Section III is an extensive chart of organisms and their classic features including former names, the antimicrobic test method to be used, drugs of choice for empiric therapy, and other interesting caveats and bits of information. Selecting and administering a therapeutic regimen is the job of the clinician, and this chart does not recommend therapy; instead, it informs the laboratorians of the potential therapeutic choices a physician may have. More detailed therapeutic information is available elsewhere (39, 66). Unfortunately, nomenclature and taxonomy are moving targets and genus or species names often change quickly. Even so, some nomenclature changes may not translate into practice quickly, while others may. The *Companion* is not a reference for determining taxonomic position; therefore, the reader should refer to the literature or to updated resources similar to the website at www.bacterio.cict.fr/index.html, "List of Prokaryotic names with Standing in Nomenclature." Other websites from which updated information, particularly regarding viruses and parasites, was obtained for these charts include the Centers for Disease Control and Prevention site at www.cdc.gov. Information on yeasts and fungi was taken from the Doctor Fungus website at www.doctorfungus.com, and the descriptions and susceptibility data are used with permission. Serology information sources are available elsewhere in more detail (29), but salient points are listed in the charts.

To use *all* of the algorithms effectively, you will need access to the following reagents and supplies: catalase, oxidase, 6.5% NaCl broth, pyrrolidonyl arylamidase (PYR) disks, leucine aminopeptidase (LAP) disks, esculin, vancomycin disks, glucose OF (oxidative-fermentative medium) tubes, triple sugar iron (TSI) slants, acid-fast bacillus (AFB) stain, motility medium, xylose or trehalose broth, phenylalanine slants, sucrose broth, polymyxin B disk, indole reagent, urea slant, nitrate broth, mannitol broth, lysine decarboxylase, lactose broth, maltose broth, X/V disks or strips, buffered charcoal-yeast extract (BCYE) medium for *Legionella*, and brain heart infusion (BHI) broth with serum. Whether or not you elect to use all of the tables is strictly up to you. In addition, some of the components may be read from your automated instrument results, but it is necessary to use caution and judgment when doing so.

Organism	Extent of ID/Comments
Gram-positive rods	Accept confidence reports of 90% or greater but confirm with colony morphology and susceptibility tests. Do not rely on these tests for fastidious isolates. Refer to reference labs. See Flowchart 1.
Gram-positive cocci	Accept confidence reports of 90% or greater but confirm with colony and susceptibility test observations. No automated system is highly accurate with viridans group streptococci; resist identifying them by automated methods until the literature demonstrates a significant degree of accuracy. See Flowchart 2.
Gram-negative diplococci, oxidase positive	Confidence values of 90% or greater should be observed. If not, use a backup method. DNA probes or amplification methods may be best for *Neisseria gonorrhoeae*, except in cases of abuse. See Flowchart 3.
Anaerobes	See Flowcharts 4 and 5.
Gram-negative rods or coccobacilli, oxidase negative ("enterics")	Accept a report from the identification instrument or method if it gives 95% or greater confidence. If less than 95%, consider a backup method to confirm the results unless they are confirmed by morphology and susceptibility tests. See Flowchart 6.
Gram-negative coccobacilli or rods, oxidase positive (nonfermenters or fastidious organisms)	For nonfermenters, accept a report of 85% confidence or greater. If less than 85%, repeat with a backup method. If still not confident in the result, consult and use special media or refer out for identification. Identification results for very fastidious isolates may be incorrect. See Flowcharts 7, 8, and 9.

Algorithms for the Identification of Organisms

Flowcharts are modified from the eighth edition of the *Manual of Clinical Microbiology.*

All laboratorians would like easy-to-use instruments or simple identification algorithms that lead quickly to the correct species to report. Until a few years ago, the limited number of species we considered significant in the laboratory allowed for that kind of decision tree. With the advent of molecular genetics and the ease with which a taxon can be fully evaluated, the number of new genera and species we confront on a daily basis has exploded, making classic algorithms more difficult to prepare and even more burdensome to interpret. In this regard, these algorithms are modified from the eighth and ninth editions of the *Manual of Clinical Microbiology* and presented as "yes (positive) or no (negative)" responses. Decision trees such as these must be used along with other tests and our interpretive judgment and can rarely stand alone as completely accurate identification methods. At best, they only help us think through to the next step or the next decision and perhaps lead us to rule out certain organisms.

Bacteria

Flowchart 1. Aerobic, gram-positive rods

Flowchart 2. Gram-positive cocci in clusters and groups

Flowchart 3. Gram-positive cocci in pairs and chains (catalase negative)

Flowchart 4. Anaerobes: rods

Flowchart 5. Anaerobes: cocci

Flowchart 6. Gram-negative rods that grow well on blood agar, including glucose fermenters

Flowchart 7. Glucose nonfermenters that grow well on blood agar

Flowchart 8. Oxidase-positive, non-glucose-fermenting gram-negative rods

Flowchart 9. Gram-negative rods with poor or no growth on blood agar

Fungi

Flowchart 10. Mycology

Parasitology

Flowchart 11. Intestinal amoebae

Flowchart 12. Intestinal flagellates

Flowchart 13. Helminth eggs

Abbreviations used in the flowcharts are as follows: AFB, acid-fast bacilli; AM, ampicillin; BBE, *Bacteroides*-bile esculin agar; BCYE, buffered charcoal-yeast extract medium; BHI, brain heart infusion medium; CDC, Centers for Disease Control and Prevention; LAP, leucine aminopeptidase; MAC, MacConkey agar; OF, oxidative-fermentative medium; ONPG, *o*-nitrophenyl-β-D-galactopyranoside; PYR, pyrrolidonyl arylamidase; R, resistant; S, susceptible; TSI, triple sugar iron agar; X/V, growth factors for *Haemophilus* organisms.

Note: In the flowcharts, a horizontal arrow indicates a "yes" or "positive" response, and a vertical arrow indicates a "no" or "negative" response.

Flowchart 1

Aerobic, gram-positive rods

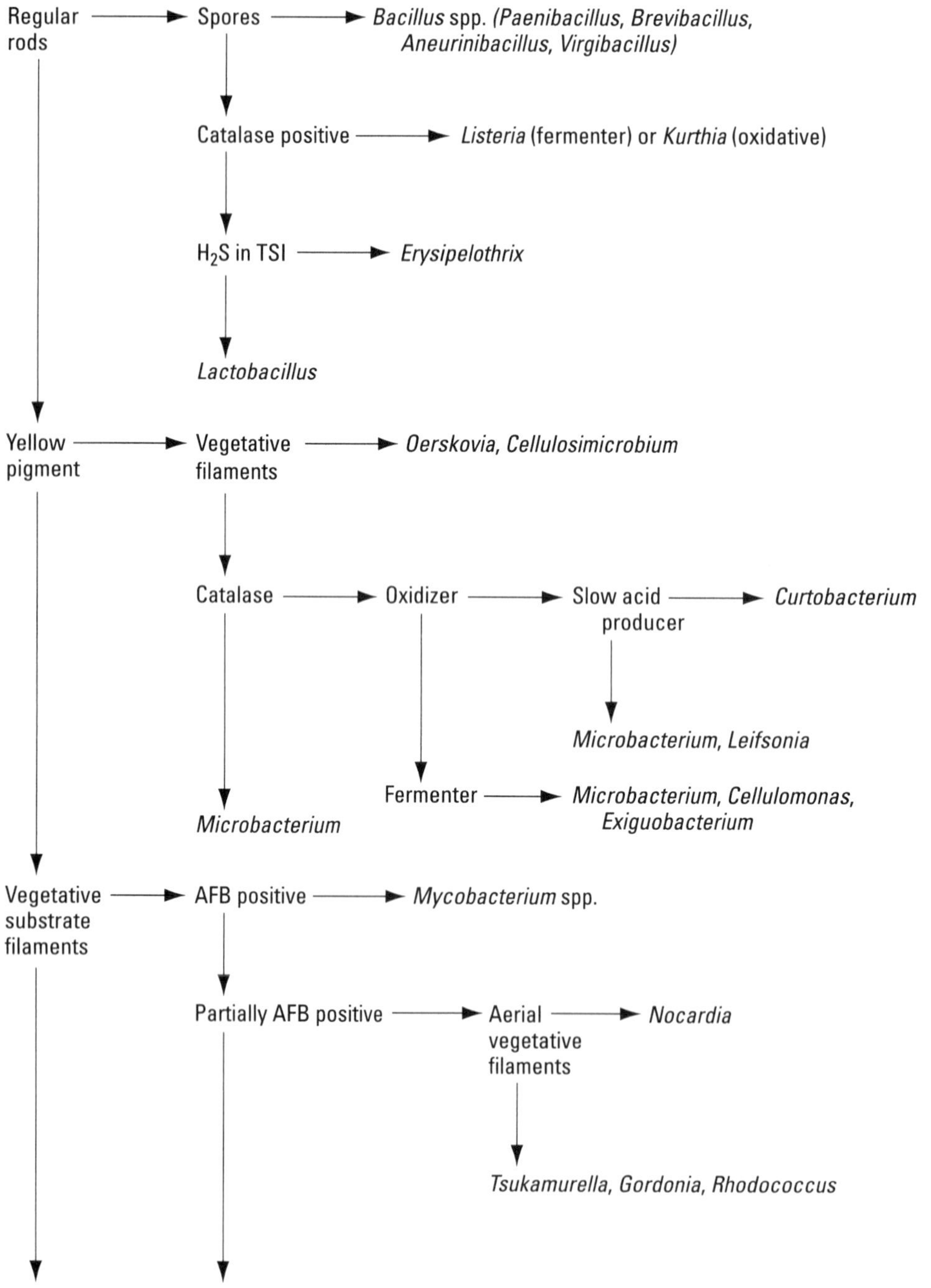
Regular rods
Spores
Bacillus spp. *(Paenibacillus, Brevibacillus, Aneurinibacillus, Virgibacillus)*
Catalase positive
Listeria (fermenter) or *Kurthia* (oxidative)
H_2S in TSI
Erysipelothrix
Lactobacillus
Yellow pigment
Vegetative filaments
Oerskovia, Cellulosimicrobium
Catalase
Oxidizer
Slow acid producer
Curtobacterium
Microbacterium, Leifsonia
Fermenter
Microbacterium, Cellulomonas, Exiguobacterium
Microbacterium
Vegetative substrate filaments
AFB positive
Mycobacterium spp.
Partially AFB positive
Aerial vegetative filaments
Nocardia
Tsukamurella, Gordonia, Rhodococcus

(continued)

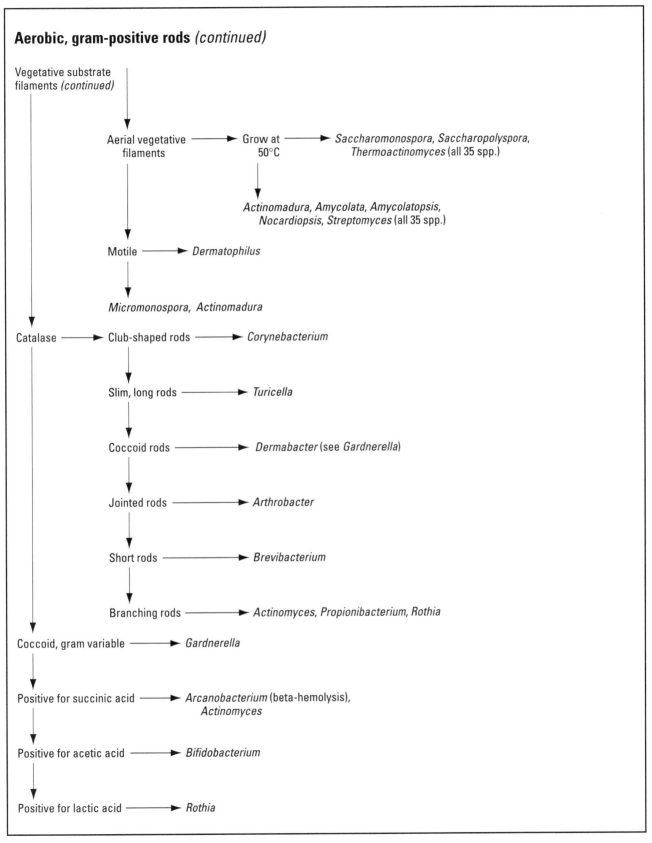

Aerobic, gram-positive rods *(continued)*

Vegetative substrate filaments *(continued)*

- ↓ Aerial vegetative filaments → Grow at 50°C → *Saccharomonospora*, *Saccharopolyspora*, *Thermoactinomyces* (all 35 spp.)
  - ↓ (from Grow at 50°C) *Actinomadura*, *Amycolata*, *Amycolatopsis*, *Nocardiopsis*, *Streptomyces* (all 35 spp.)
- ↓ Motile → *Dermatophilus*
- ↓ *Micromonospora*, *Actinomadura*

↓

Catalase → Club-shaped rods → *Corynebacterium*

- ↓ Slim, long rods → *Turicella*
- ↓ Coccoid rods → *Dermabacter* (see *Gardnerella*)
- ↓ Jointed rods → *Arthrobacter*
- ↓ Short rods → *Brevibacterium*
- ↓ Branching rods → *Actinomyces*, *Propionibacterium*, *Rothia*

↓

Coccoid, gram variable → *Gardnerella*

↓

Positive for succinic acid → *Arcanobacterium* (beta-hemolysis), *Actinomyces*

↓

Positive for acetic acid → *Bifidobacterium*

↓

Positive for lactic acid → *Rothia*

Flowchart 2

Gram-positive cocci in clusters and groups

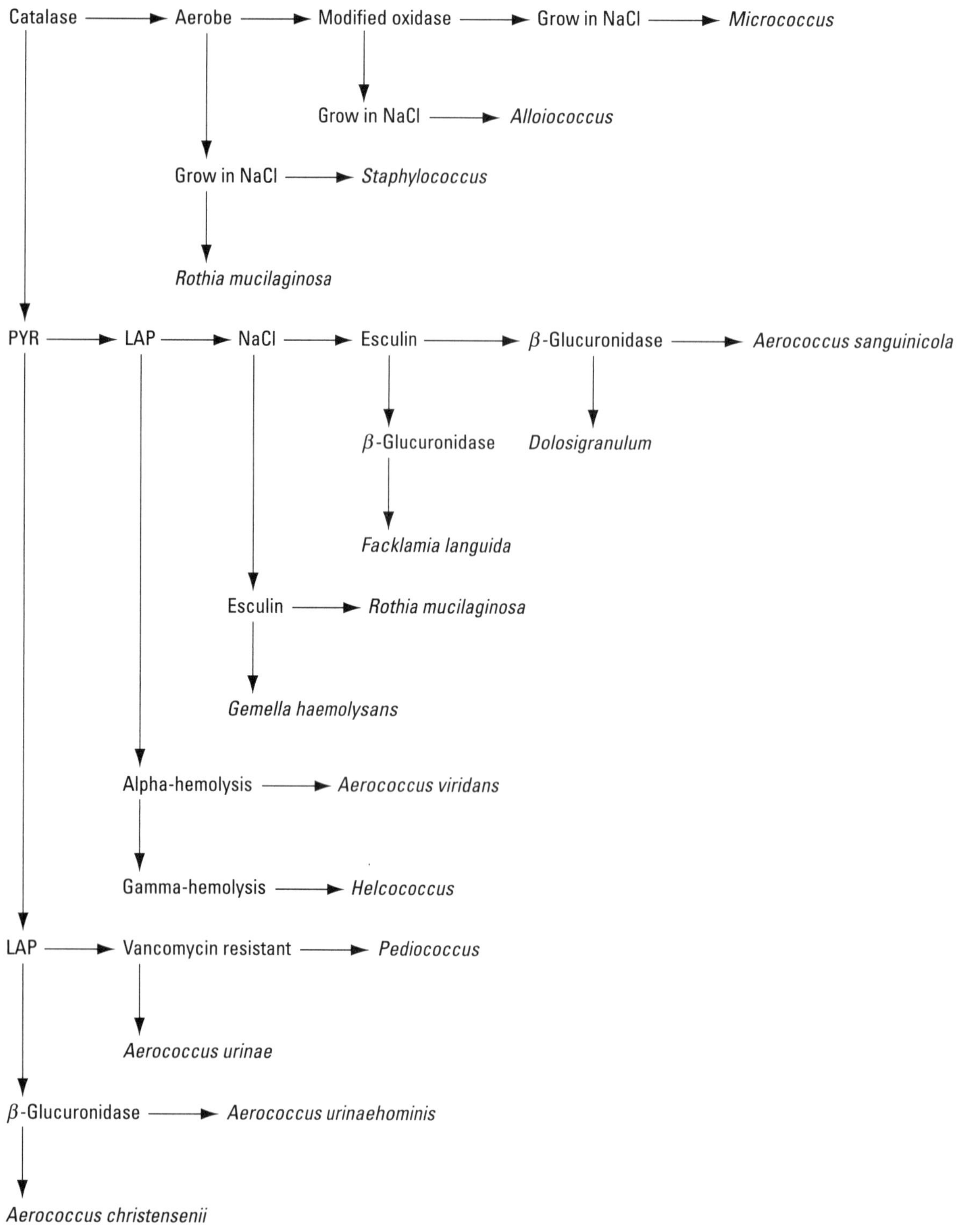

Catalase
Aerobe
Modified oxidase
Grow in NaCl
Micrococcus
Grow in NaCl
Alloiococcus
Grow in NaCl
Staphylococcus
Rothia mucilaginosa
PYR
LAP
NaCl
Esculin
β-Glucuronidase
Aerococcus sanguinicola
β-Glucuronidase
Dolosigranulum
Facklamia languida
Esculin
Rothia mucilaginosa
Gemella haemolysans
Alpha-hemolysis
Aerococcus viridans
Gamma-hemolysis
Helcococcus
LAP
Vancomycin resistant
Pediococcus
Aerococcus urinae
β-Glucuronidase
Aerococcus urinaehominis
Aerococcus christensenii

Flowchart 3

Gram-positive cocci in pairs and chains (catalase negative)

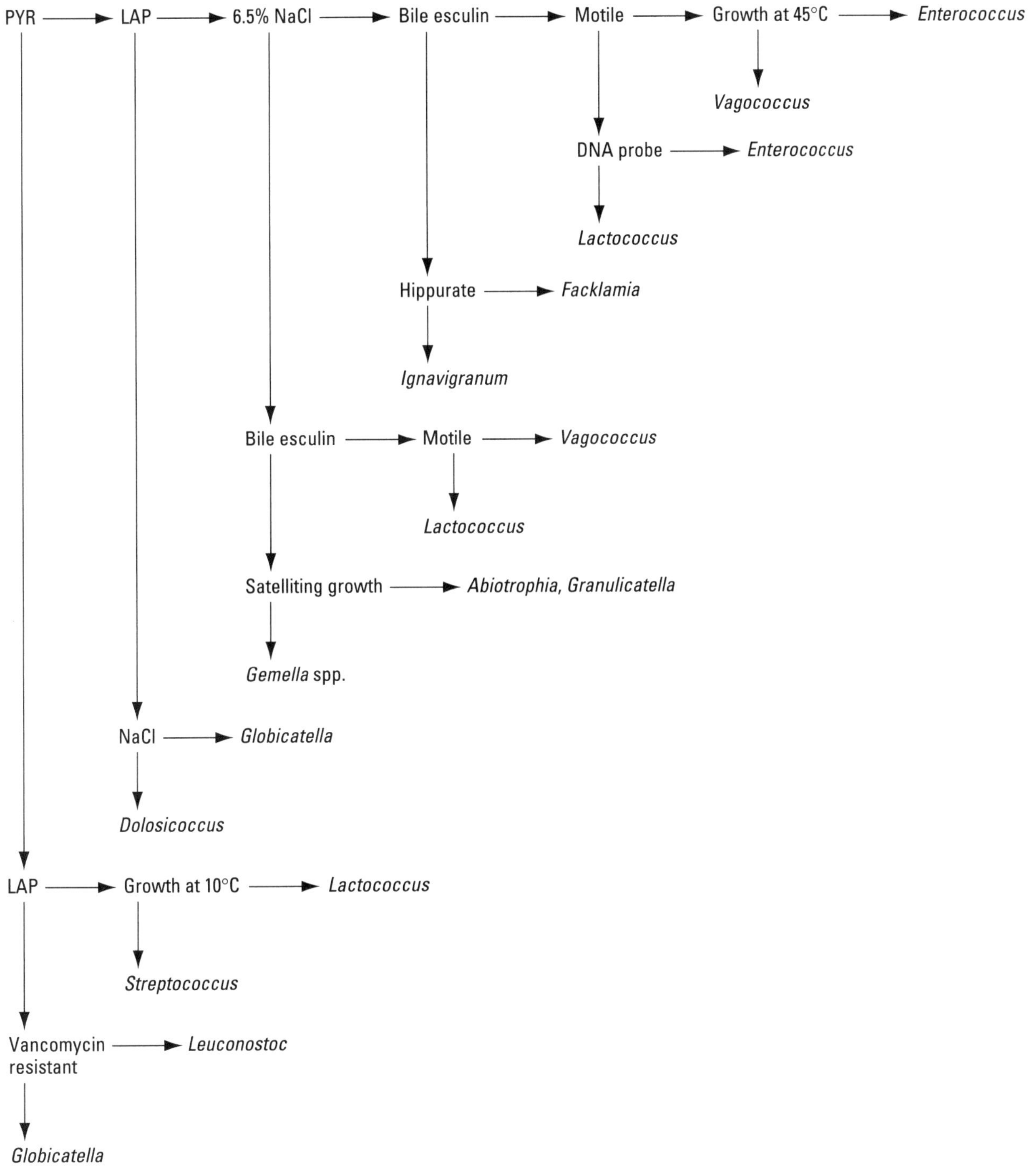
PYR
LAP
6.5% NaCl
Bile esculin
Motile
Growth at 45°C
Enterococcus
Vagococcus
DNA probe
Enterococcus
Lactococcus
Hippurate
Facklamia
Ignavigranum
Bile esculin
Motile
Vagococcus
Lactococcus
Satelliting growth
Abiotrophia, Granulicatella
Gemella spp.
NaCl
Globicatella
Dolosicoccus
LAP
Growth at 10°C
Lactococcus
Streptococcus
Vancomycin resistant
Leuconostoc
Globicatella

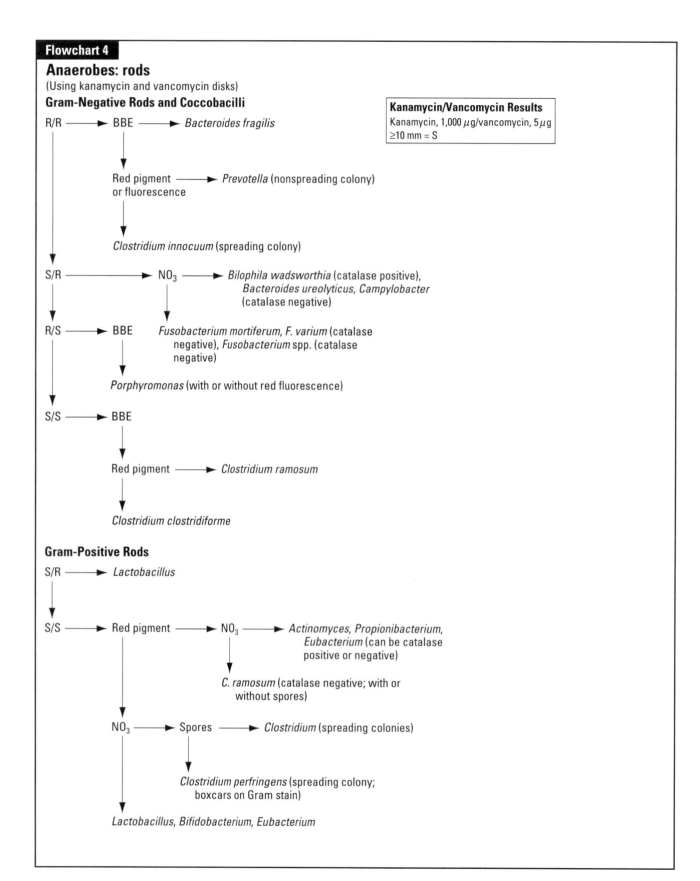

Flowchart 4

Anaerobes: rods

(Using kanamycin and vancomycin disks)

Kanamycin/Vancomycin Results
Kanamycin, 1,000 μg/vancomycin, 5 μg
$\geq$10 mm = S

Gram-Negative Rods and Coccobacilli

R/R → BBE → *Bacteroides fragilis*

- BBE ↓ Red pigment or fluorescence → *Prevotella* (nonspreading colony)
- Red pigment or fluorescence ↓ *Clostridium innocuum* (spreading colony)

R/R ↓ S/R → NO_3 → *Bilophila wadsworthia* (catalase positive), *Bacteroides ureolyticus, Campylobacter* (catalase negative)

- NO_3 ↓ *Fusobacterium mortiferum, F. varium* (catalase negative), *Fusobacterium* spp. (catalase negative)

S/R ↓ R/S → BBE

- BBE ↓ *Porphyromonas* (with or without red fluorescence)

R/S ↓ S/S → BBE

- BBE ↓ Red pigment → *Clostridium ramosum*
- Red pigment ↓ *Clostridium clostridiforme*

Gram-Positive Rods

S/R → *Lactobacillus*

S/R ↓ S/S → Red pigment → NO_3 → *Actinomyces, Propionibacterium, Eubacterium* (can be catalase positive or negative)

- NO_3 ↓ *C. ramosum* (catalase negative; with or without spores)
- Red pigment ↓ NO_3 → Spores → *Clostridium* (spreading colonies)
  - Spores ↓ *Clostridium perfringens* (spreading colony; boxcars on Gram stain)
  - NO_3 ↓ *Lactobacillus, Bifidobacterium, Eubacterium*

Flowchart 5

Anaerobes: cocci

(Using kanamycin and vancomycin disks)

Kanamycin/Vancomycin Results
Kanamycin, 1,000 μg/vancomycin, 5 μg
$\geq$10 mm = S

Gram-positive coccus → S/S → *Peptostreptococcus* (anaerobic gram-positive cocci)

Gram-negative coccus → S/R → *Veillonella*, *Acidaminococcus*, *Megasphaera*

Flowchart 6

Gram-negative rods that grow well on blood agar, including glucose fermenters

(Recent taxonomic changes are discussed in reference 63a and may not be reflected here)

Rods

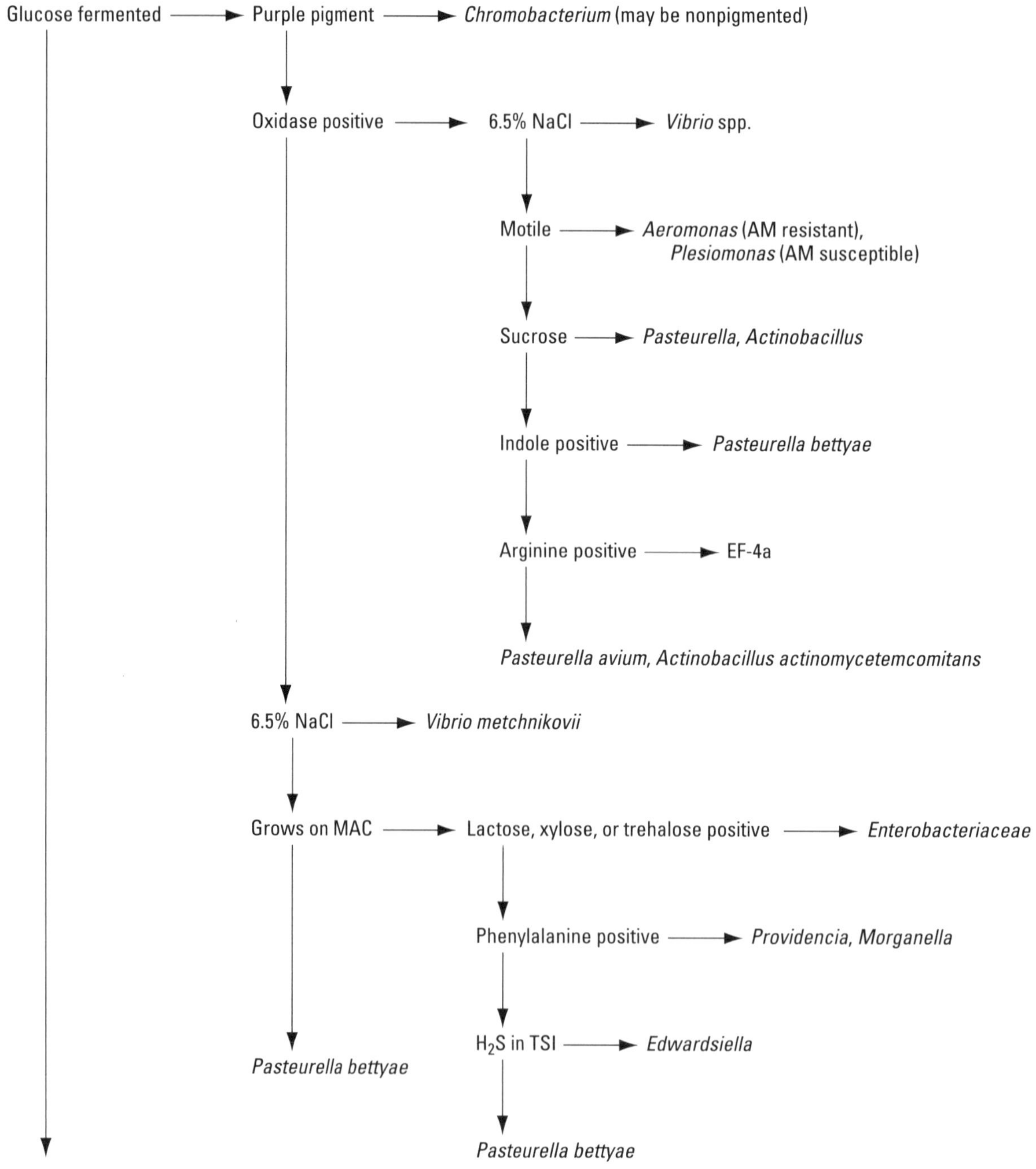

Glucose fermented
Purple pigment
Chromobacterium (may be nonpigmented)
Oxidase positive
6.5% NaCl
Vibrio spp.
Motile
Aeromonas (AM resistant),
Plesiomonas (AM susceptible)
Sucrose
Pasteurella, *Actinobacillus*
Indole positive
Pasteurella bettyae
Arginine positive
EF-4a
Pasteurella avium, *Actinobacillus actinomycetemcomitans*
6.5% NaCl
Vibrio metchnikovii
Grows on MAC
Lactose, xylose, or trehalose positive
Enterobacteriaceae
Phenylalanine positive
Providencia, *Morganella*
H_2S in TSI
Edwardsiella
Pasteurella bettyae
Pasteurella bettyae

(continued)

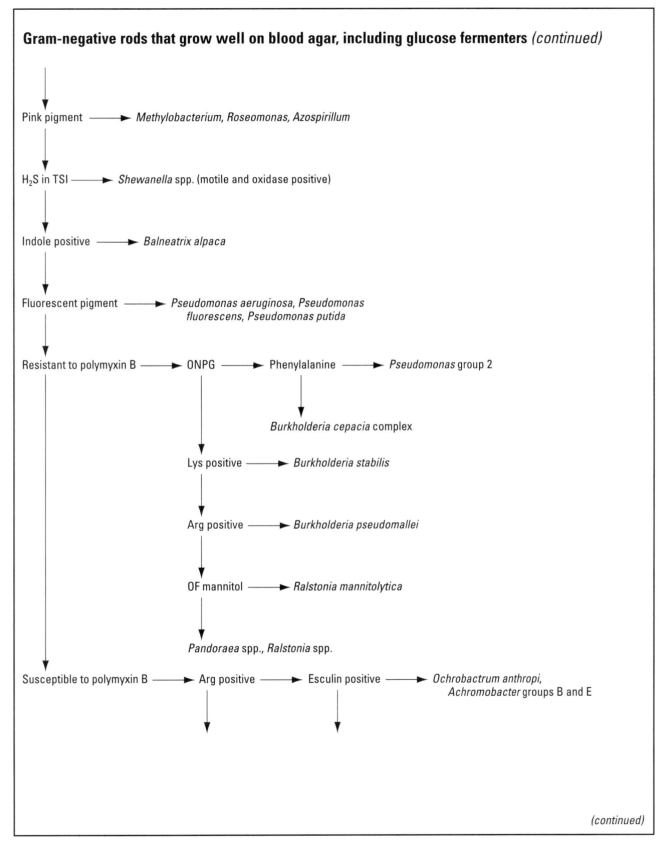

Gram-negative rods that grow well on blood agar, including glucose fermenters *(continued)*

- Pink pigment → *Methylobacterium, Roseomonas, Azospirillum*
- H_2S in TSI → *Shewanella* spp. (motile and oxidase positive)
- Indole positive → *Balneatrix alpaca*
- Fluorescent pigment → *Pseudomonas aeruginosa, Pseudomonas fluorescens, Pseudomonas putida*
- Resistant to polymyxin B → ONPG → Phenylalanine → *Pseudomonas* group 2
  - Phenylalanine ↓ *Burkholderia cepacia* complex
  - ONPG ↓ Lys positive → *Burkholderia stabilis*
    - ↓ Arg positive → *Burkholderia pseudomallei*
    - ↓ OF mannitol → *Ralstonia mannitolytica*
    - ↓ *Pandoraea* spp., *Ralstonia* spp.
- Susceptible to polymyxin B → Arg positive → Esculin positive → *Ochrobactrum anthropi, Achromobacter* groups B and E
  - Arg positive ↓
  - Esculin positive ↓

(continued)

Gram-negative rods that grow well on blood agar, including glucose fermenters *(continued)*

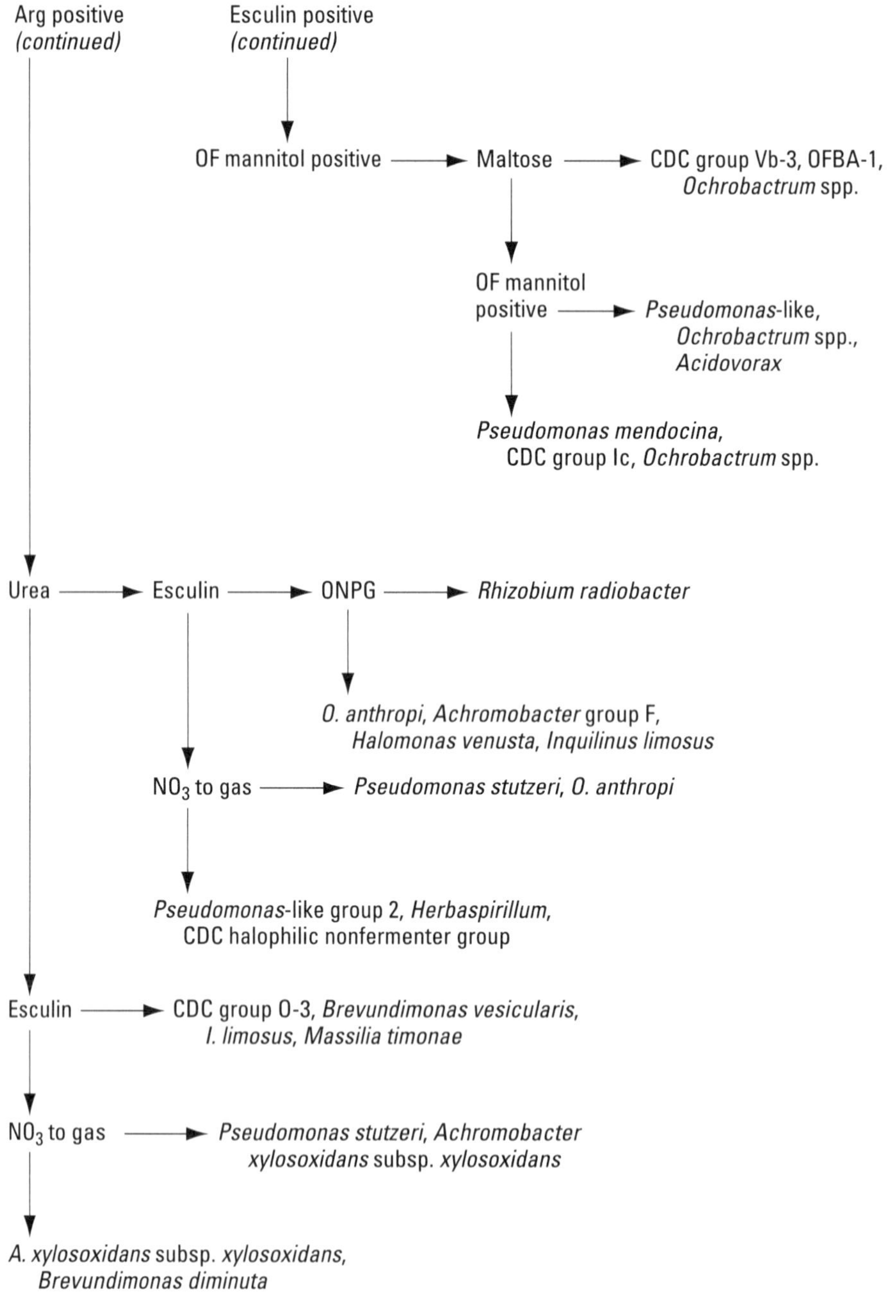
Arg positive (continued)
Esculin positive (continued)
OF mannitol positive
Maltose
CDC group Vb-3, OFBA-1, Ochrobactrum spp.
OF mannitol positive
Pseudomonas-like, Ochrobactrum spp., Acidovorax
Pseudomonas mendocina, CDC group Ic, Ochrobactrum spp.
Urea
Esculin
ONPG
Rhizobium radiobacter
O. anthropi, Achromobacter group F, Halomonas venusta, Inquilinus limosus
NO3 to gas
Pseudomonas stutzeri, O. anthropi
Pseudomonas-like group 2, Herbaspirillum, CDC halophilic nonfermenter group
Esculin
CDC group O-3, Brevundimonas vesicularis, I. limosus, Massilia timonae
NO3 to gas
Pseudomonas stutzeri, Achromobacter xylosoxidans subsp. xylosoxidans
A. xylosoxidans subsp. xylosoxidans, Brevundimonas diminuta

Flowchart 7

Glucose nonfermenters that grow well on blood agar

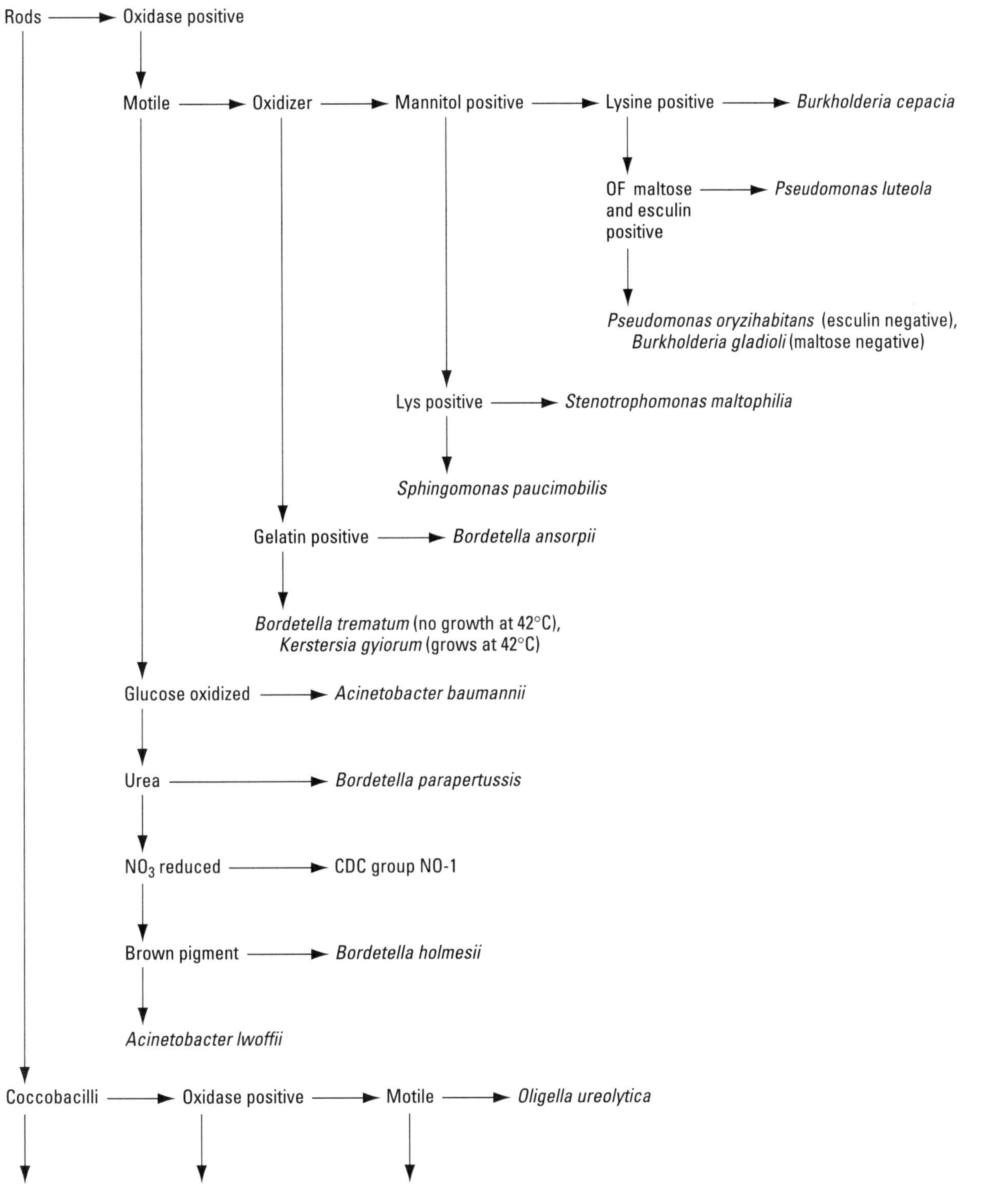
Rods
Oxidase positive
Motile
Oxidizer
Mannitol positive
Lysine positive
Burkholderia cepacia
OF maltose and esculin positive
Pseudomonas luteola
Pseudomonas oryzihabitans (esculin negative), Burkholderia gladioli (maltose negative)
Lys positive
Stenotrophomonas maltophilia
Sphingomonas paucimobilis
Gelatin positive
Bordetella ansorpii
Bordetella trematum (no growth at 42°C), Kerstersia gyiorum (grows at 42°C)
Glucose oxidized
Acinetobacter baumannii
Urea
Bordetella parapertussis
NO3 reduced
CDC group NO-1
Brown pigment
Bordetella holmesii
Acinetobacter lwoffii
Coccobacilli
Oxidase positive
Motile
Oligella ureolytica

(continued)

Glucose nonfermenters that grow well on blood agar *(continued)*

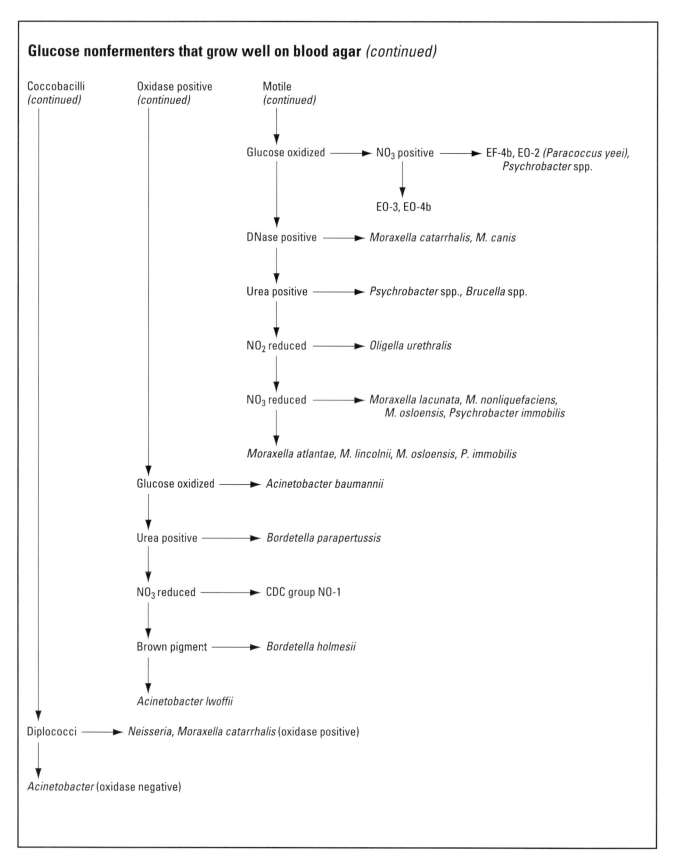

- Coccobacilli *(continued)*
  - Oxidase positive *(continued)*
    - Motile *(continued)*
      - Glucose oxidized → NO_3 positive → EF-4b, EO-2 *(Paracoccus yeei)*, *Psychrobacter* spp.
        - ↓ EO-3, EO-4b
      - ↓ DNase positive → *Moraxella catarrhalis, M. canis*
      - ↓ Urea positive → *Psychrobacter* spp., *Brucella* spp.
      - ↓ NO_2 reduced → *Oligella urethralis*
      - ↓ NO_3 reduced → *Moraxella lacunata, M. nonliquefaciens, M. osloensis, Psychrobacter immobilis*
      - ↓ *Moraxella atlantae, M. lincolnii, M. osloensis, P. immobilis*
    - ↓ Glucose oxidized → *Acinetobacter baumannii*
    - ↓ Urea positive → *Bordetella parapertussis*
    - ↓ NO_3 reduced → CDC group NO-1
    - ↓ Brown pigment → *Bordetella holmesii*
    - ↓ *Acinetobacter lwoffii*
- ↓ Diplococci → *Neisseria, Moraxella catarrhalis* (oxidase positive)
- ↓ *Acinetobacter* (oxidase negative)

Flowchart 8

Oxidase-positive, non-glucose-fermenting gram-negative rods

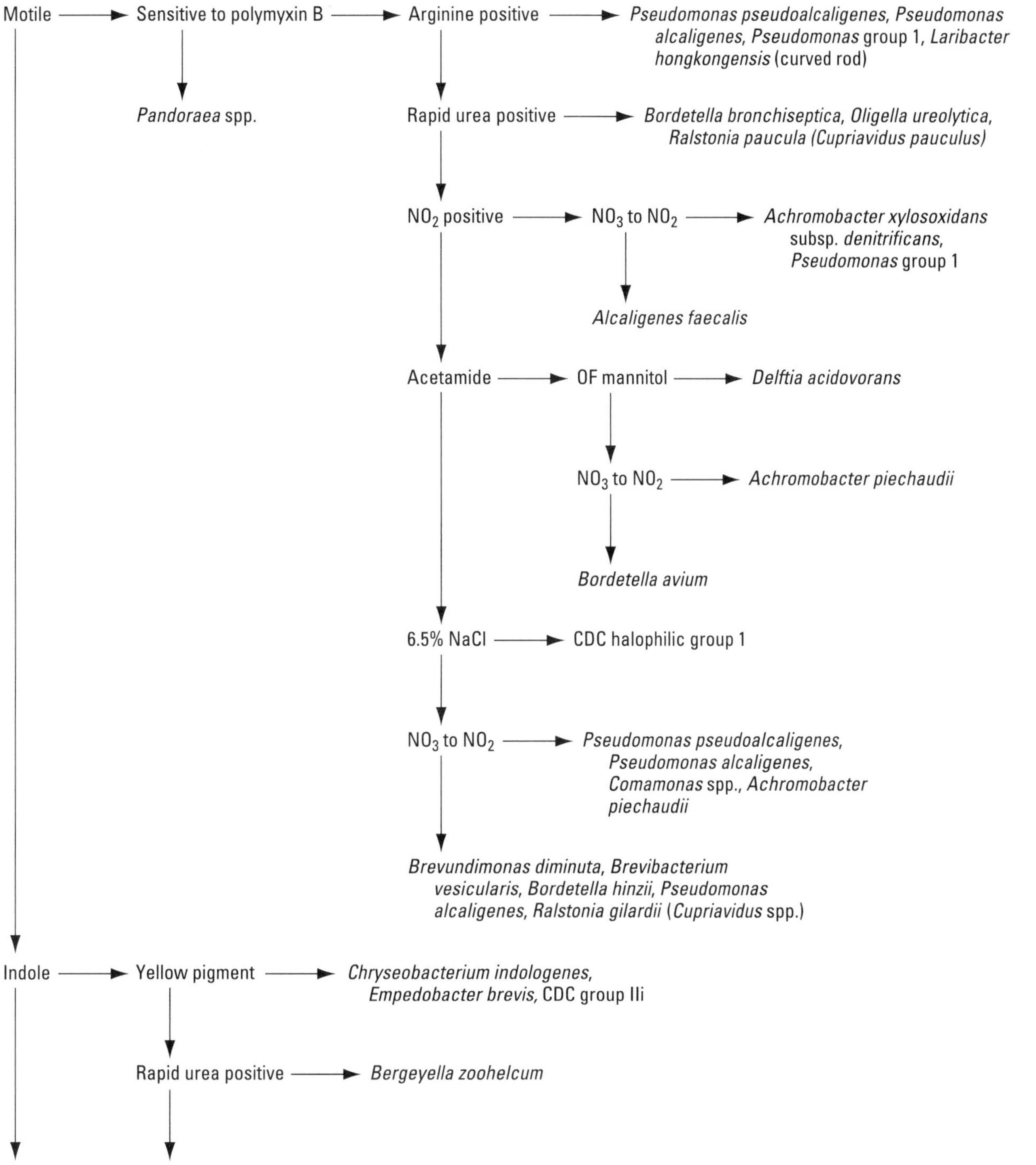

Motile
Sensitive to polymyxin B
Arginine positive
Pseudomonas pseudoalcaligenes, *Pseudomonas alcaligenes*, *Pseudomonas* group 1, *Laribacter hongkongensis* (curved rod)
Pandoraea spp.
Rapid urea positive
Bordetella bronchiseptica, *Oligella ureolytica*, *Ralstonia paucula (Cupriavidus pauculus)*
NO_2 positive
NO_3 to NO_2
Achromobacter xylosoxidans subsp. *denitrificans*, *Pseudomonas* group 1
Alcaligenes faecalis
Acetamide
OF mannitol
Delftia acidovorans
NO_3 to NO_2
Achromobacter piechaudii
Bordetella avium
6.5% NaCl
CDC halophilic group 1
NO_3 to NO_2
Pseudomonas pseudoalcaligenes, *Pseudomonas alcaligenes*, *Comamonas* spp., *Achromobacter piechaudii*
Brevundimonas diminuta, *Brevibacterium vesicularis*, *Bordetella hinzii*, *Pseudomonas alcaligenes*, *Ralstonia gilardii* (*Cupriavidus* spp.)
Indole
Yellow pigment
Chryseobacterium indologenes, *Empedobacter brevis,* CDC group IIi
Rapid urea positive
Bergeyella zoohelcum

(continued)

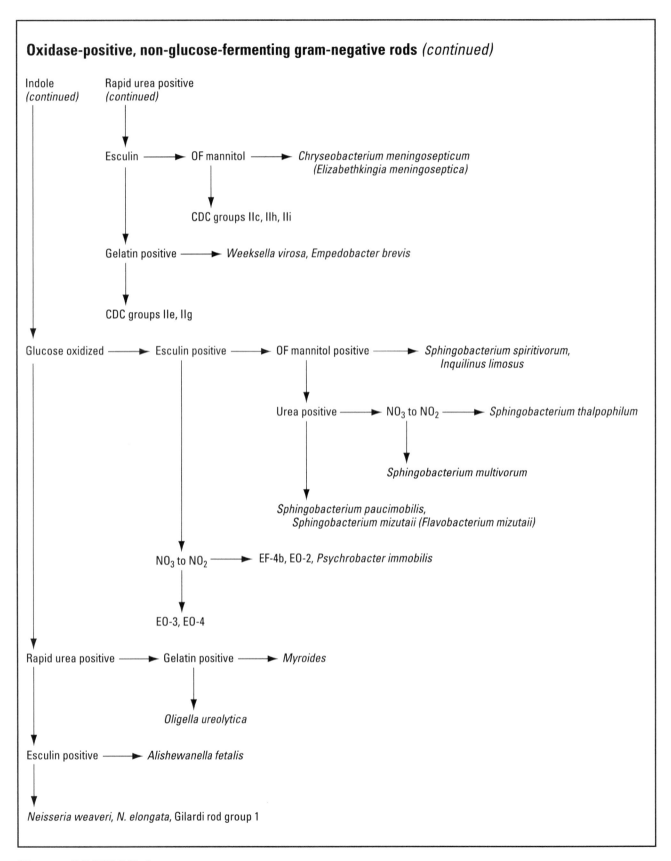

Oxidase-positive, non-glucose-fermenting gram-negative rods *(continued)*

Indole *(continued)*

- Rapid urea positive *(continued)*
  - Esculin → OF mannitol → *Chryseobacterium meningosepticum (Elizabethkingia meningoseptica)*
    - ↓ OF mannitol: CDC groups IIc, IIh, IIi
  - ↓ Esculin: Gelatin positive → *Weeksella virosa*, *Empedobacter brevis*
    - ↓ Gelatin: CDC groups IIe, IIg
- ↓ Indole: Glucose oxidized → Esculin positive → OF mannitol positive → *Sphingobacterium spiritivorum*, *Inquilinus limosus*
  - ↓ OF mannitol: Urea positive → NO_3 to NO_2 → *Sphingobacterium thalpophilum*
    - ↓ NO_3 to NO_2: *Sphingobacterium multivorum*
    - ↓ Urea: *Sphingobacterium paucimobilis*, *Sphingobacterium mizutaii (Flavobacterium mizutaii)*
  - ↓ Esculin positive: NO_3 to NO_2 → EF-4b, EO-2, *Psychrobacter immobilis*
    - ↓ NO_3 to NO_2: EO-3, EO-4
- ↓ Glucose oxidized: Rapid urea positive → Gelatin positive → *Myroides*
  - ↓ Gelatin positive: *Oligella ureolytica*
  - ↓ Rapid urea positive: Esculin positive → *Alishewanella fetalis*
    - ↓ Esculin positive: *Neisseria weaveri*, *N. elongata*, Gilardi rod group 1

Flowchart 9

Gram-negative rods with poor or no growth on blood agar

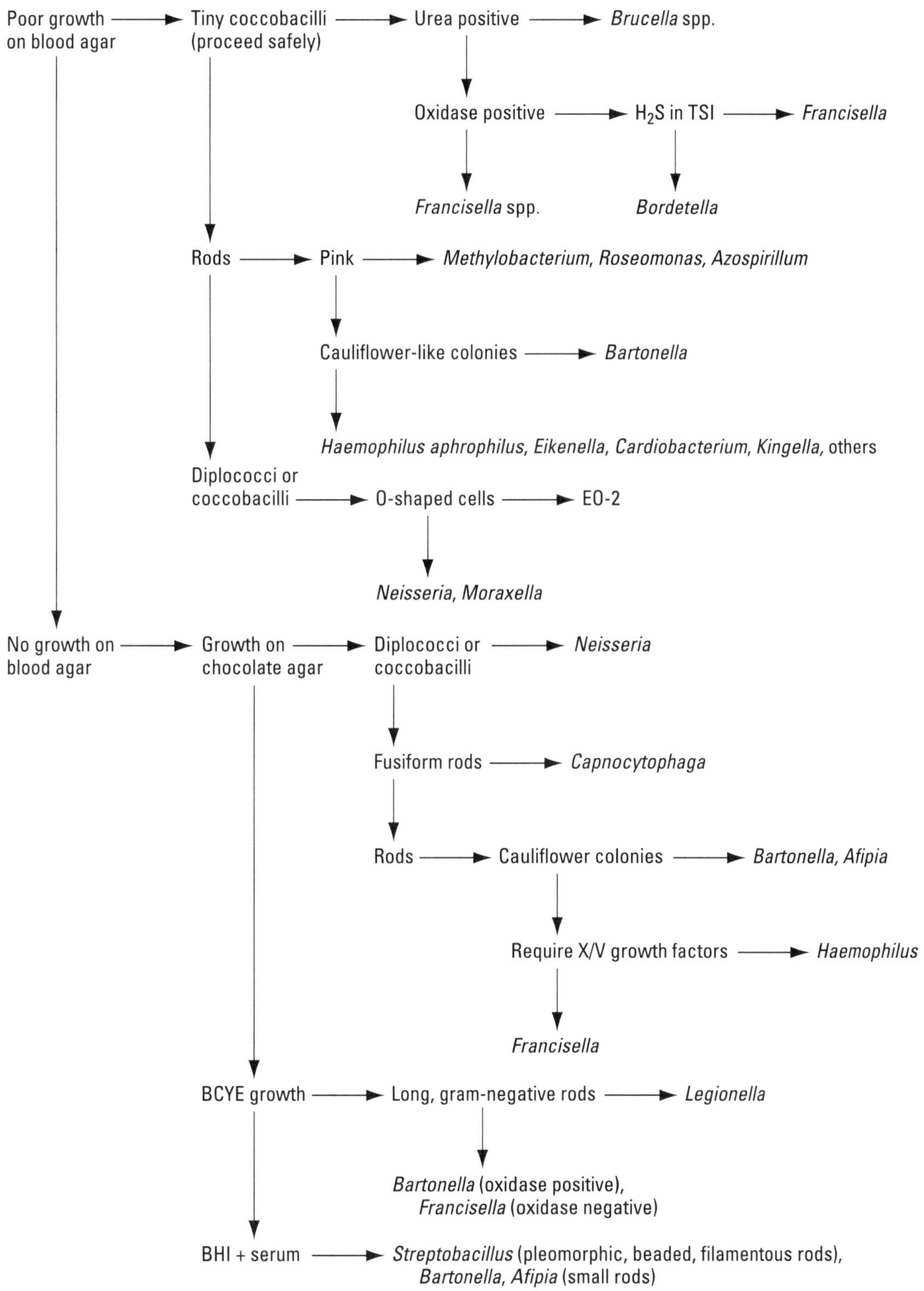
Poor growth on blood agar
Tiny coccobacilli (proceed safely)
Urea positive
Brucella spp.
Oxidase positive
H_2S in TSI
Francisella
Francisella spp.
Bordetella
Rods
Pink
Methylobacterium, Roseomonas, Azospirillum
Cauliflower-like colonies
Bartonella
Haemophilus aphrophilus, Eikenella, Cardiobacterium, Kingella, others
Diplococci or coccobacilli
O-shaped cells
EO-2
Neisseria, Moraxella
No growth on blood agar
Growth on chocolate agar
Diplococci or coccobacilli
Neisseria
Fusiform rods
Capnocytophaga
Rods
Cauliflower colonies
Bartonella, Afipia
Require X/V growth factors
Haemophilus
Francisella
BCYE growth
Long, gram-negative rods
Legionella
Bartonella (oxidase positive), *Francisella* (oxidase negative)
BHI + serum
Streptobacillus (pleomorphic, beaded, filamentous rods), *Bartonella, Afipia* (small rods)

Flowchart 10

Mycology

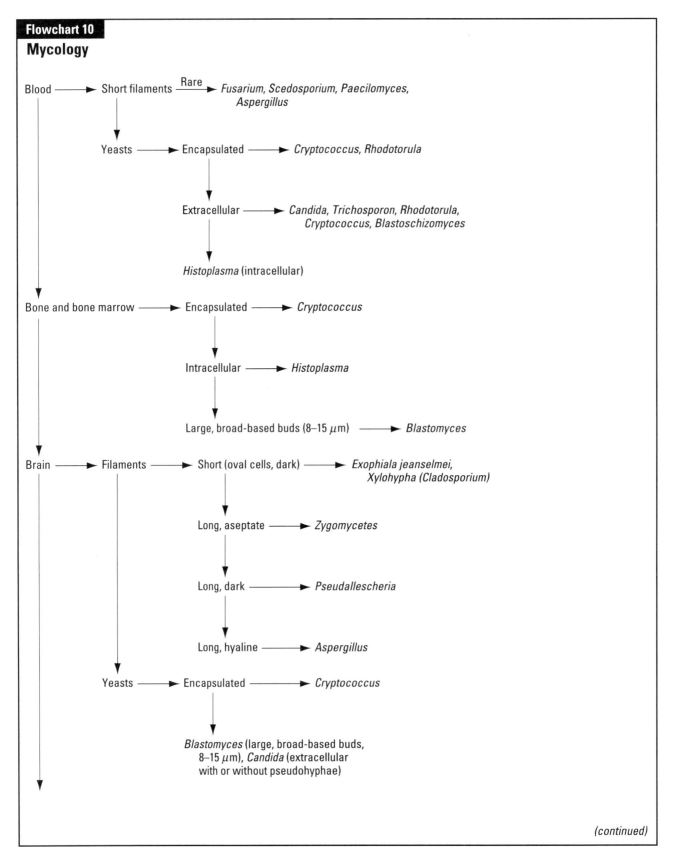

- Blood
  - Short filaments → (Rare) → *Fusarium, Scedosporium, Paecilomyces, Aspergillus*
  - Yeasts
    - Encapsulated → *Cryptococcus, Rhodotorula*
    - Extracellular → *Candida, Trichosporon, Rhodotorula, Cryptococcus, Blastoschizomyces*
    - *Histoplasma* (intracellular)
- Bone and bone marrow
  - Encapsulated → *Cryptococcus*
  - Intracellular → *Histoplasma*
  - Large, broad-based buds (8–15 μm) → *Blastomyces*
- Brain
  - Filaments
    - Short (oval cells, dark) → *Exophiala jeanselmei, Xylohypha (Cladosporium)*
    - Long, aseptate → *Zygomycetes*
    - Long, dark → *Pseudallescheria*
    - Long, hyaline → *Aspergillus*
  - Yeasts
    - Encapsulated → *Cryptococcus*
    - *Blastomyces* (large, broad-based buds, 8–15 μm), *Candida* (extracellular with or without pseudohyphae)

(continued)

Mycology *(continued)*

Bronchial lavage, wash, sputum → Yeasts → *Cryptococcus* (encapsulated); *Histoplasma*, *Penicillium marneffei* (intracellular); *Blastomyces* (large, broad-based buds); *Paracoccidioides* (multiple buds, narrow base); *Saccharomyces*, *Candida* (extracellular with or without pseudohyphae)

septate → *Absidia*, *Rhizopus*, *Mucor*

tate → *Aspergillus*, *Fusarium*, *Geotrichum*, *Paecilomyces*

→ *Trichosporon*, *Aspergillus*, *Pseudallescheria*

apsulated → *Cryptococcus*, *Rhodotorula*

nencapsulated → *Candida*, *Rhodotorula*

racellular → *Histoplasma*

m) → *Coccidioides*

Aspergillus, *Fusarium*, *Acremonium*, *Arthrographis*

ndida

Aspergillus

Candida

(continued)

Mycology *(continued)*

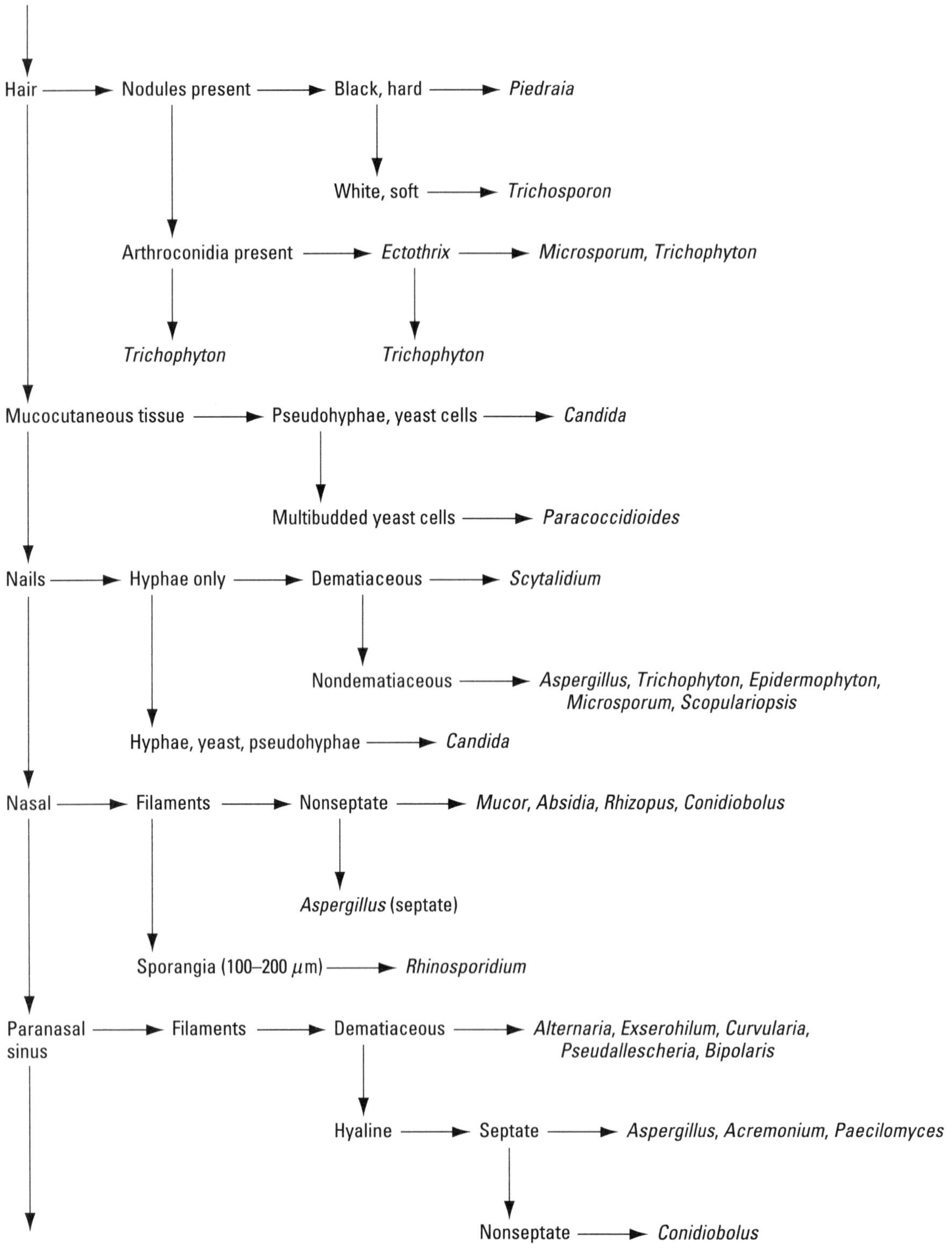
Hair
Nodules present
Black, hard
Piedraia
White, soft
Trichosporon
Arthroconidia present
Ectothrix
Microsporum, Trichophyton
Trichophyton
Trichophyton
Mucocutaneous tissue
Pseudohyphae, yeast cells
Candida
Multibudded yeast cells
Paracoccidioides
Nails
Hyphae only
Dematiaceous
Scytalidium
Nondematiaceous
Aspergillus, Trichophyton, Epidermophyton, Microsporum, Scopulariopsis
Hyphae, yeast, pseudohyphae
Candida
Nasal
Filaments
Nonseptate
Mucor, Absidia, Rhizopus, Conidiobolus
Aspergillus (septate)
Sporangia (100–200 μm)
Rhinosporidium
Paranasal sinus
Filaments
Dematiaceous
Alternaria, Exserohilum, Curvularia, Pseudallescheria, Bipolaris
Hyaline
Septate
Aspergillus, Acremonium, Paecilomyces
Nonseptate
Conidiobolus

(continued)

Mycology *(continued)*

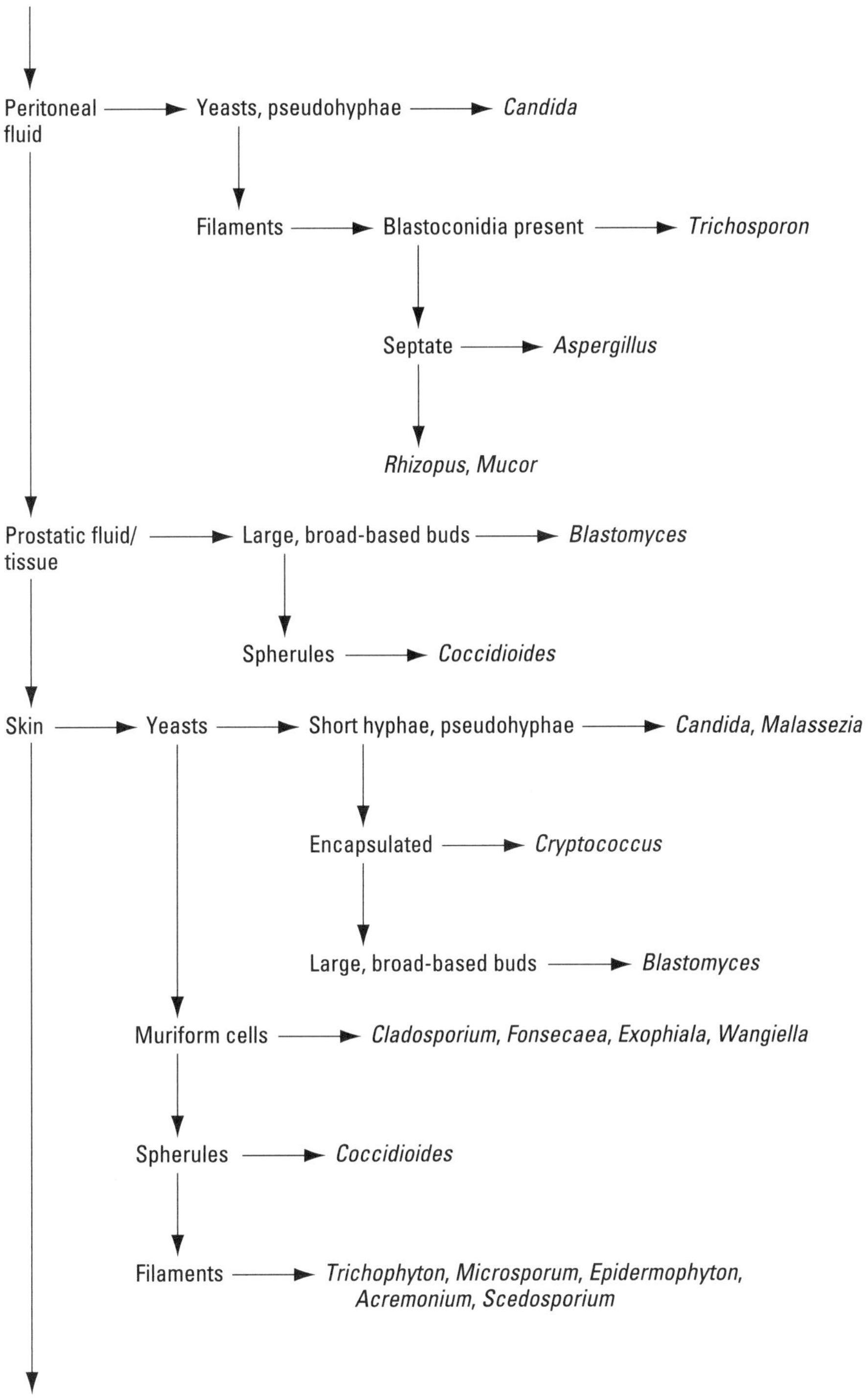
Peritoneal fluid
Yeasts, pseudohyphae
Candida
Filaments
Blastoconidia present
Trichosporon
Septate
Aspergillus
Rhizopus, Mucor
Prostatic fluid/ tissue
Large, broad-based buds
Blastomyces
Spherules
Coccidioides
Skin
Yeasts
Short hyphae, pseudohyphae
Candida, Malassezia
Encapsulated
Cryptococcus
Large, broad-based buds
Blastomyces
Muriform cells
Cladosporium, Fonsecaea, Exophiala, Wangiella
Spherules
Coccidioides
Filaments
Trichophyton, Microsporum, Epidermophyton, Acremonium, Scedosporium

(continued)

Mycology *(continued)*

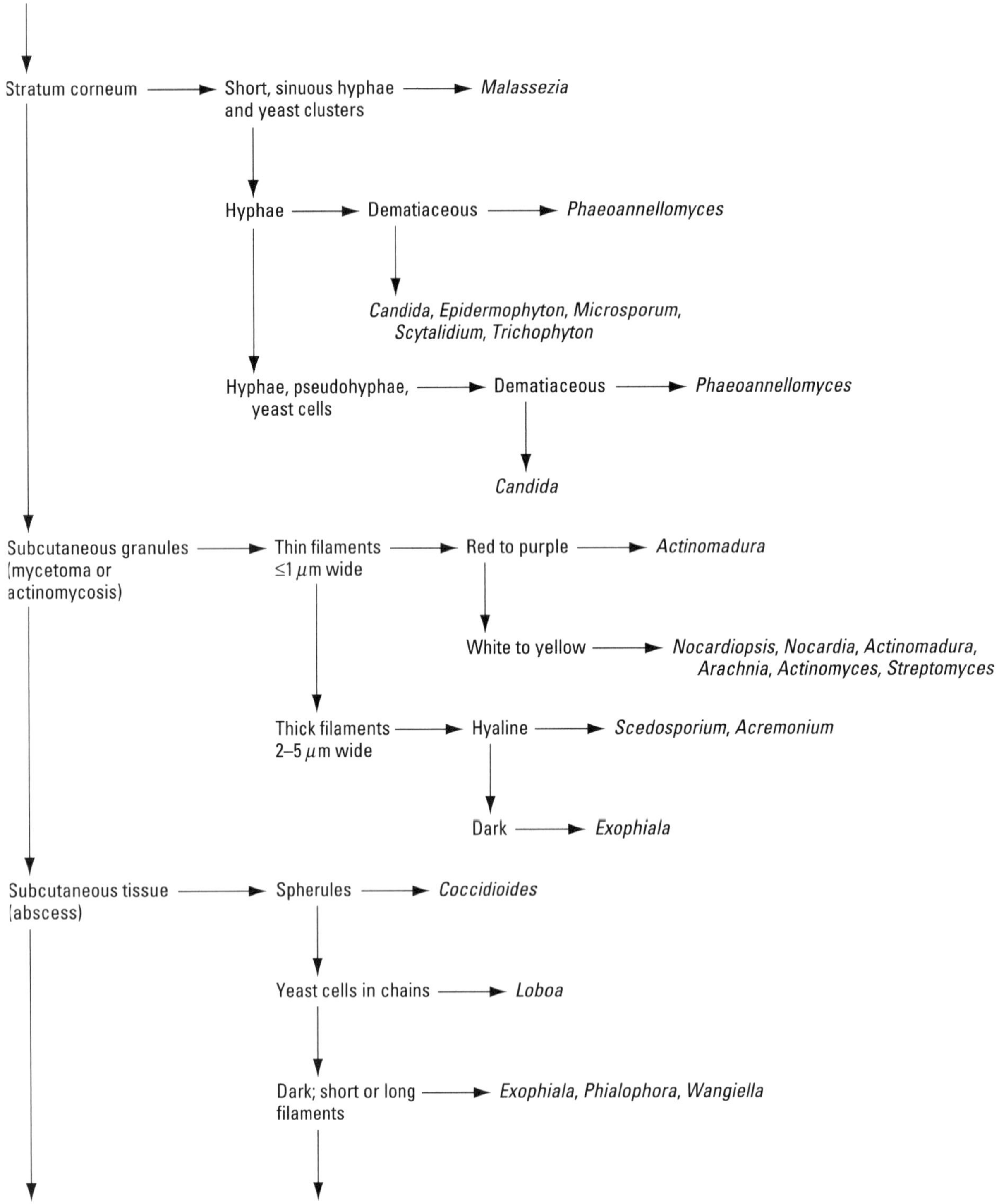
Stratum corneum
Short, sinuous hyphae and yeast clusters
Malassezia
Hyphae
Dematiaceous
Phaeoannellomyces
Candida, Epidermophyton, Microsporum, Scytalidium, Trichophyton
Hyphae, pseudohyphae, yeast cells
Dematiaceous
Phaeoannellomyces
Candida
Subcutaneous granules (mycetoma or actinomycosis)
Thin filaments ≤1 μm wide
Red to purple
Actinomadura
White to yellow
Nocardiopsis, Nocardia, Actinomadura, Arachnia, Actinomyces, Streptomyces
Thick filaments 2–5 μm wide
Hyaline
Scedosporium, Acremonium
Dark
Exophiala
Subcutaneous tissue (abscess)
Spherules
Coccidioides
Yeast cells in chains
Loboa
Dark; short or long filaments
Exophiala, Phialophora, Wangiella

(continued)

Mycology *(continued)*

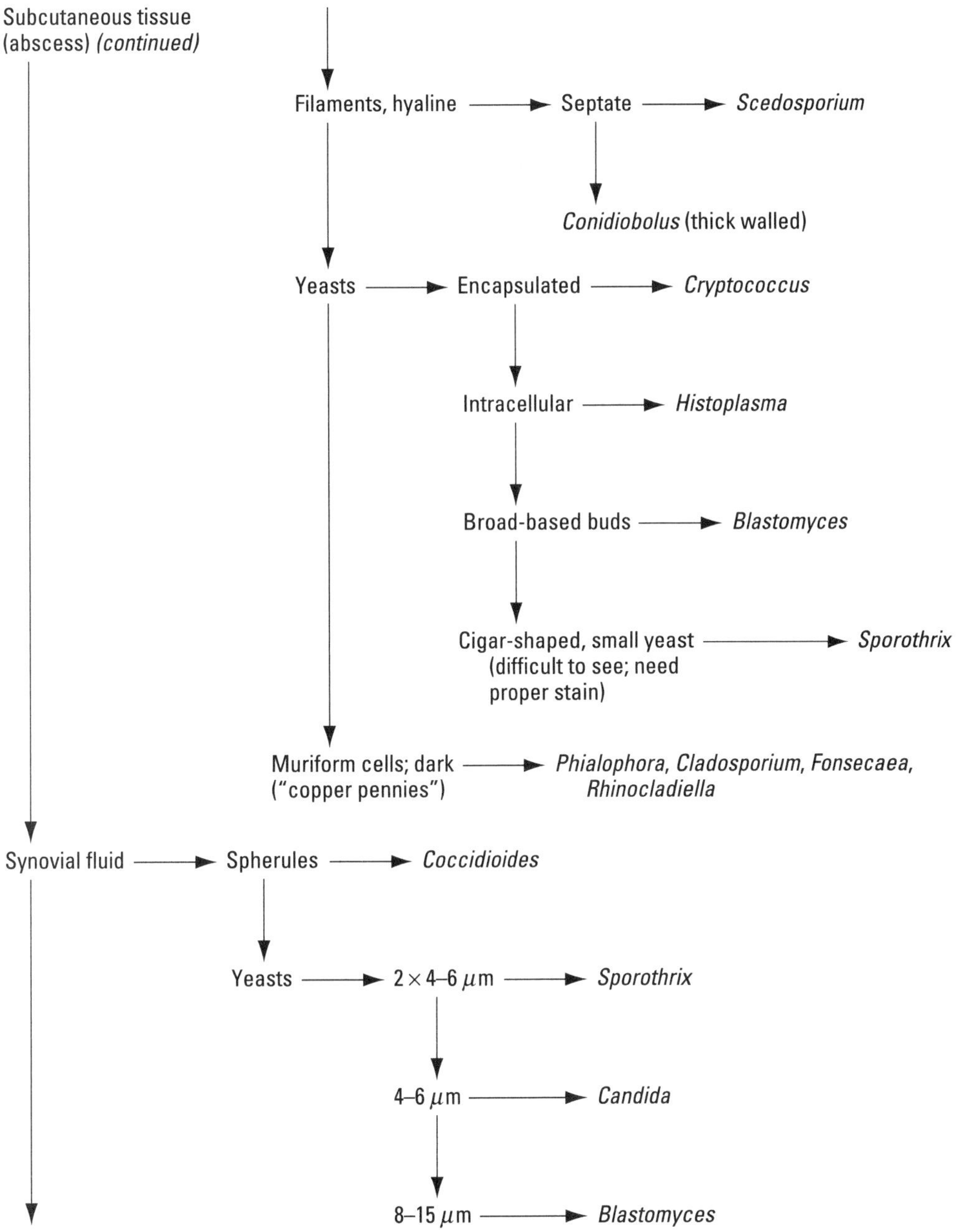
Subcutaneous tissue (abscess) (continued)
Filaments, hyaline
Septate
Scedosporium
Conidiobolus (thick walled)
Yeasts
Encapsulated
Cryptococcus
Intracellular
Histoplasma
Broad-based buds
Blastomyces
Cigar-shaped, small yeast (difficult to see; need proper stain)
Sporothrix
Muriform cells; dark ("copper pennies")
Phialophora, Cladosporium, Fonsecaea, Rhinocladiella
Synovial fluid
Spherules
Coccidioides
Yeasts
2 × 4–6 μm
Sporothrix
4–6 μm
Candida
8–15 μm
Blastomyces

(continued)

Mycology *(continued)*

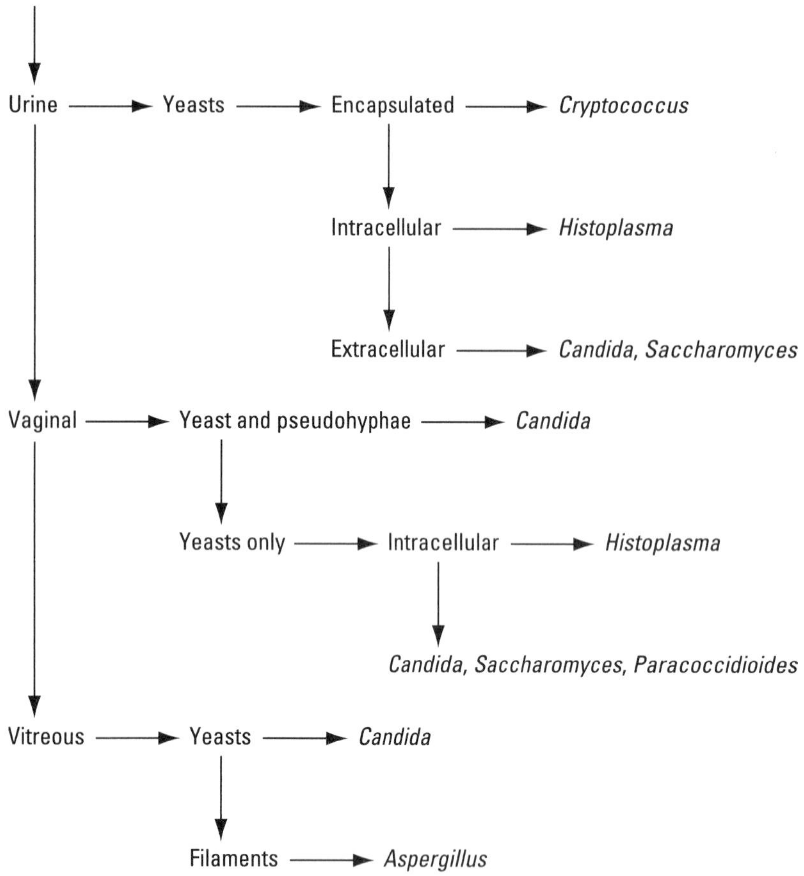

Urine
Yeasts
Encapsulated
Cryptococcus
Intracellular
Histoplasma
Extracellular
Candida, Saccharomyces
Vaginal
Yeast and pseudohyphae
Candida
Yeasts only
Intracellular
Histoplasma
Candida, Saccharomyces, Paracoccidioides
Vitreous
Yeasts
Candida
Filaments
Aspergillus

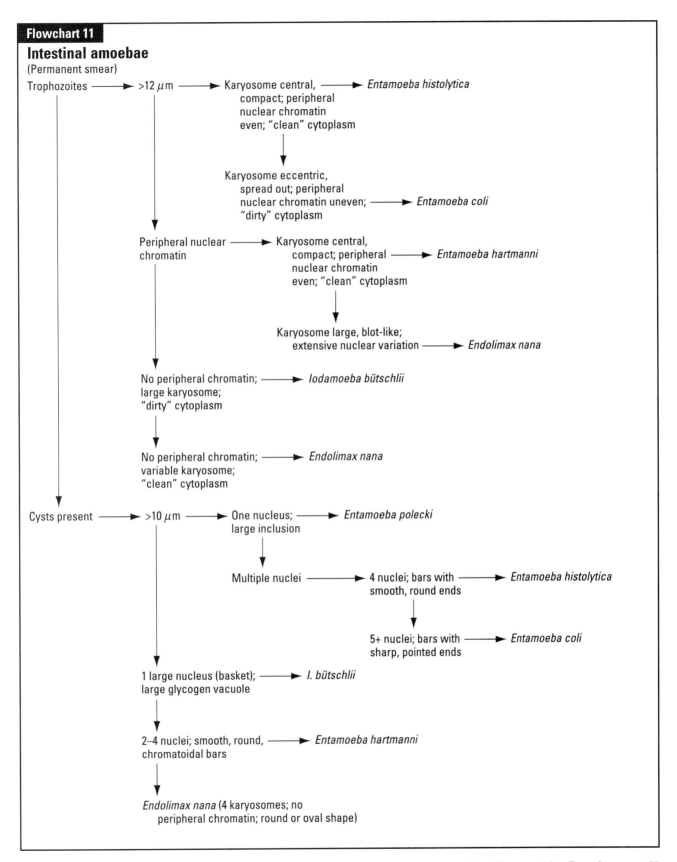

Flowchart 11

Intestinal amoebae

(Permanent smear)

- Trophozoites →
  - >12 μm →
    - Karyosome central, compact; peripheral nuclear chromatin even; "clean" cytoplasm → *Entamoeba histolytica*
    - ↓ Karyosome eccentric, spread out; peripheral nuclear chromatin uneven; "dirty" cytoplasm → *Entamoeba coli*
  - ↓ Peripheral nuclear chromatin →
    - Karyosome central, compact; peripheral nuclear chromatin even; "clean" cytoplasm → *Entamoeba hartmanni*
    - ↓ Karyosome large, blot-like; extensive nuclear variation → *Endolimax nana*
  - ↓ No peripheral chromatin; large karyosome; "dirty" cytoplasm → *Iodamoeba bütschlii*
  - ↓ No peripheral chromatin; variable karyosome; "clean" cytoplasm → *Endolimax nana*
- ↓ Cysts present →
  - >10 μm →
    - One nucleus; large inclusion → *Entamoeba polecki*
    - ↓ Multiple nuclei →
      - 4 nuclei; bars with smooth, round ends → *Entamoeba histolytica*
      - ↓ 5+ nuclei; bars with sharp, pointed ends → *Entamoeba coli*
  - ↓ 1 large nucleus (basket); large glycogen vacuole → *I. bütschlii*
  - ↓ 2–4 nuclei; smooth, round, chromatoidal bars → *Entamoeba hartmanni*
  - ↓ *Endolimax nana* (4 karyosomes; no peripheral chromatin; round or oval shape)

Flowchart 12

Intestinal flagellates

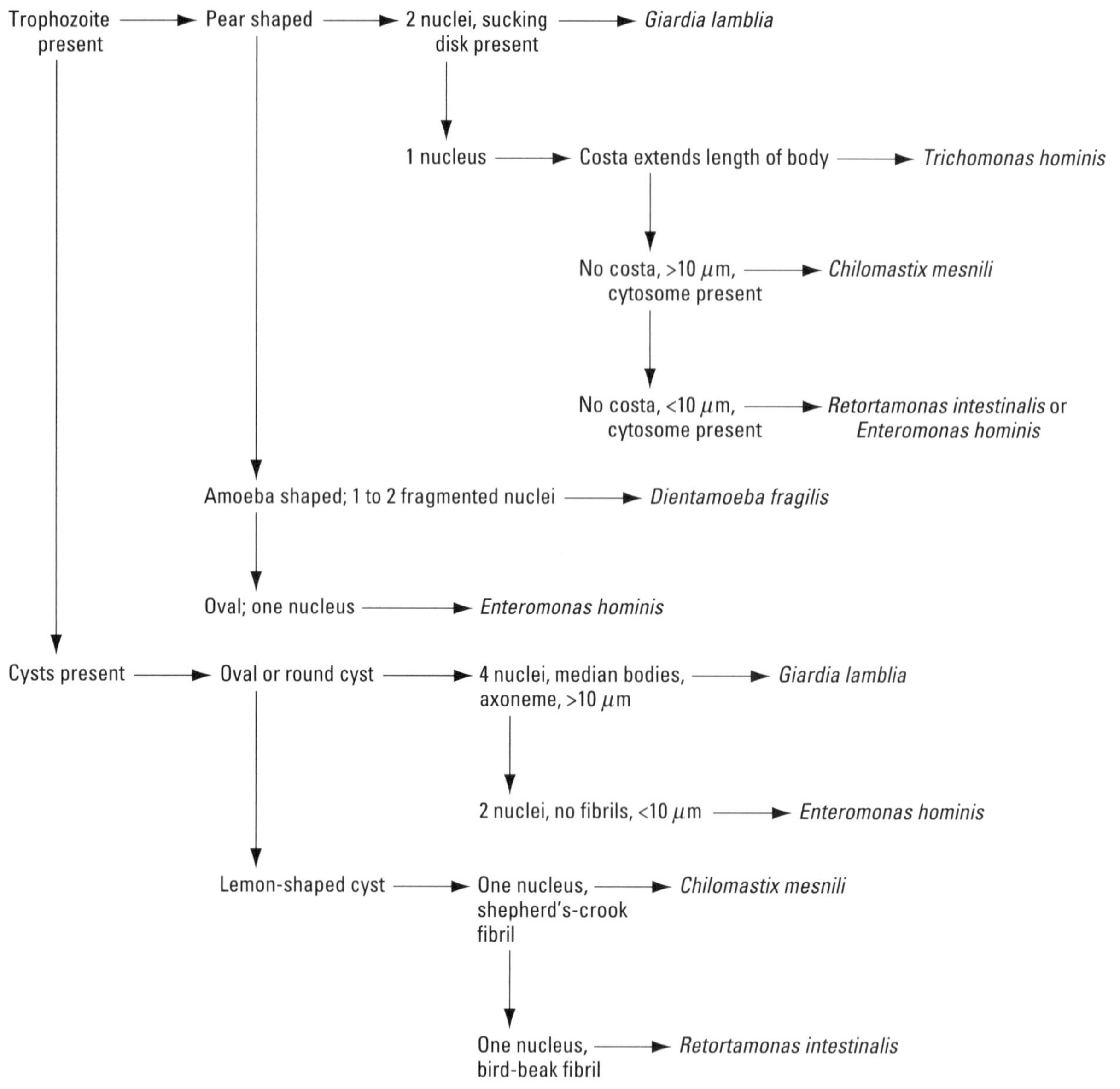
Trophozoite present
Pear shaped
2 nuclei, sucking disk present
Giardia lamblia
1 nucleus
Costa extends length of body
Trichomonas hominis
No costa, >10 μm, cytosome present
Chilomastix mesnili
No costa, <10 μm, cytosome present
Retortamonas intestinalis or Enteromonas hominis
Amoeba shaped; 1 to 2 fragmented nuclei
Dientamoeba fragilis
Oval; one nucleus
Enteromonas hominis
Cysts present
Oval or round cyst
4 nuclei, median bodies, axoneme, >10 μm
Giardia lamblia
2 nuclei, no fibrils, <10 μm
Enteromonas hominis
Lemon-shaped cyst
One nucleus, shepherd's-crook fibril
Chilomastix mesnili
One nucleus, bird-beak fibril
Retortamonas intestinalis

Flowchart 13

Helminth eggs

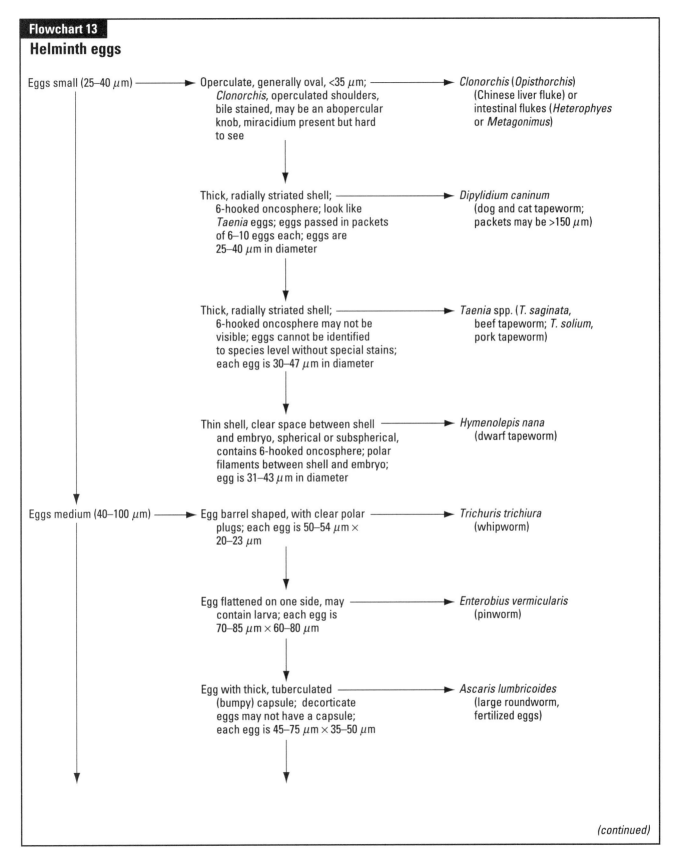

Egg size	Description	Identification
Eggs small (25–40 μm)	Operculate, generally oval, <35 μm; *Clonorchis*, operculated shoulders, bile stained, may be an abopercular knob, miracidium present but hard to see	*Clonorchis* (*Opisthorchis*) (Chinese liver fluke) or intestinal flukes (*Heterophyes* or *Metagonimus*)
	Thick, radially striated shell; 6-hooked oncosphere; look like *Taenia* eggs; eggs passed in packets of 6–10 eggs each; eggs are 25–40 μm in diameter	*Dipylidium caninum* (dog and cat tapeworm; packets may be >150 μm)
	Thick, radially striated shell; 6-hooked oncosphere may not be visible; eggs cannot be identified to species level without special stains; each egg is 30–47 μm in diameter	*Taenia* spp. (*T. saginata*, beef tapeworm; *T. solium*, pork tapeworm)
	Thin shell, clear space between shell and embryo, spherical or subspherical, contains 6-hooked oncosphere; polar filaments between shell and embryo; egg is 31–43 μm in diameter	*Hymenolepis nana* (dwarf tapeworm)
Eggs medium (40–100 μm)	Egg barrel shaped, with clear polar plugs; each egg is 50–54 μm × 20–23 μm	*Trichuris trichiura* (whipworm)
	Egg flattened on one side, may contain larva; each egg is 70–85 μm × 60–80 μm	*Enterobius vermicularis* (pinworm)
	Egg with thick, tuberculated (bumpy) capsule; decorticate eggs may not have a capsule; each egg is 45–75 μm × 35–50 μm	*Ascaris lumbricoides* (large roundworm, fertilized eggs)

(continued)

Helminth eggs *(continued)*

Eggs medium (40–100 μm) *(continued)*

- Egg bluntly rounded at ends; thin shell (contains developing embryo at 8- to 16-ball stage); each egg is 56–75 μm × 36–40 μm → Hookworm
- Operculate (operculum break in shell sometimes hard to see); smooth transition from shell to operculum; small "bump" seen at abopercular end; each egg is 58–75 μm × 40–50 μm → *Diphyllobothrium latum* (broad fish tapeworm)
- Thin shell, clear space between shell and embryo; spherical; has 6-hooked oncosphere; no polar filaments; each egg is 70–85 μm × 60–80 μm → *Hymenolepis diminuta* (rat tapeworm)

Eggs large (100–180 μm) →

- Egg with opercular shoulders (looks like teapot lid and flange into which lid fits); abopercular end somewhat thick; each egg is 80–120 μm × 48–60 μm; eggs are "urn shaped" → *Paragonimus westermani* (lung fluke)
- Egg tapered at one or both ends; long thin shell containing developing embryo; each egg is 73–95 μm × 40–50 μm → *Trichostrongylus* spp.
- Egg with thick, bumpy capsule; capsule may be missing in decorticate eggs; each egg is 85–95 μm × 43–47 μm → *Ascaris lumbricoides* (large roundworm; unfertilized egg)
- Egg spined, ciliated miracidium larva may be seen; lateral spine very short; each egg is 70–100 μm × 55–65 μm → *Schistosoma japonicum* (blood fluke, stool); *S. mekongi* is smaller and rounder

(continued)

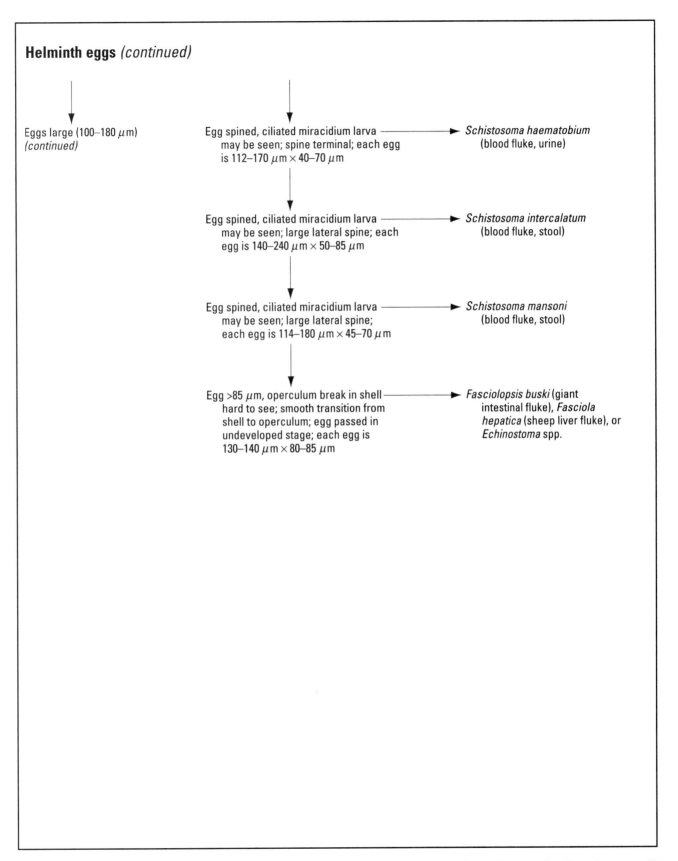

Helmint eggs *(continued)*

Eggs large (100–180 μm) *(continued)*

- Egg spined, ciliated miracidium larva may be seen; spine terminal; each egg is 112–170 μm × 40–70 μm → *Schistosoma haematobium* (blood fluke, urine)
- Egg spined, ciliated miracidium larva may be seen; large lateral spine; each egg is 140–240 μm × 50–85 μm → *Schistosoma intercalatum* (blood fluke, stool)
- Egg spined, ciliated miracidium larva may be seen; large lateral spine; each egg is 114–180 μm × 45–70 μm → *Schistosoma mansoni* (blood fluke, stool)
- Egg >85 μm, operculum break in shell hard to see; smooth transition from shell to operculum; egg passed in undeveloped stage; each egg is 130–140 μm × 80–85 μm → *Fasciolopsis buski* (giant intestinal fluke), *Fasciola hepatica* (sheep liver fluke), or *Echinostoma* spp.

SECTION II

Infectious Disease Etiology

Observations on Fastidious Isolates (Special Bacteria)

Among the "nonfermenters," rare or unusual reactions or characteristics often give clues to the identity of an isolate or provide a hint about further workup. The organisms in this chart are *not* members of the *Enterobacteriaceae*, and this chart cannot be used as a reference for final identification. It contains observations to provide some hints on what to do next.

I. Microscopic
   A. Tiny coccobacilli
      1. *Acinetobacter*
      2. *Haemophilus aphrophilus*
      3. *Actinobacillus*
      4. *Bordetella*
      5. *Brucella*
      6. *Francisella*
   B. Long, thin, wavy gram-negative rods
      1. *Capnocytophaga*: colonies on blood agar have a low, flat, spreading edge

II. Biochemical (relatively rare results from conventional tests)
   A. Indole positive
      1. *Flavobacterium* spp. and group II
      2. *Pasteurella multocida*
      3. *Cardiobacterium hominis*
      4. HB-5
      5. *Kingella indologenes*
   B. Lysine positive
      1. *Burkholderia cepacia* (oxidase positive)
      2. *Stenotrophomonas maltophilia* (oxidase negative)
   C. Ornithine positive
      1. *Eikenella corrodens*
      2. *Pasteurella multocida*

3. *Pasteurella pneumotropica*
4. *Pseudomonas putrefaciens*

D. Oxidase negative
1. *Acinetobacter* spp.
2. *Stenotrophomonas maltophilia*
3. *Chryseomonas* (VE-1), *Flavimonas* (VE-2)
4. *Capnocytophaga* and DF groups
5. *Haemophilus aphrophilus*
6. *Actinobacillus*

E. Citrate positive
1. *Acinetobacter*
2. *Ochrobactrum*
3. *Alcaligenes*
4. *Bordetella*
5. *Pseudomonas*
6. IV-C-2
7. *Chryseomonas*

F. Rapid urea (tube)
1. *Oligella* (IV-E)—instant or minutes
2. *Weeksella* (II-J)—minutes
3. *Moraxella phenylpyruvica*—minutes
4. *Brucella suis*, *B. canis*—instantly positive or within minutes (other *Brucella* spp.—overnight)

III. Colony morphology

A. Sticky, adherent colony
1. *Actinobacillus*
2. *Weeksella zoohelcum* (II-J)

B. Pitting colony
1. *Kingella kingae*
2. *Eikenella corrodens*
3. *Moraxella lacunata*

C. Spreading colony
1. *Alcaligenes faecalis*
2. *Bacillus* spp.

D. Low, flat, spreading edge
1. *Capnocytophaga*

IV. Pigment

A. Purple—*Chromobacterium violaceum* (often not pigmented)

B. Slight yellow (as seen on a swab taken from a colony)
1. *Flavobacterium meningosepticum*
2. EF-4
3. *Moraxella osloensis*
4. *Neisseria* spp. (on Loeffler's medium)

C. Deep yellow (as seen on a swab taken from a colony)
1. *Flavobacterium* spp. and group II
2. *Chryseomonas* (VE-1) and *Pseudomonas (Flavimonas)* (VE-2)

3. *Corynebacterium aquaticum*
4. *Oerskovia* spp. (gram-positive rod, smells like dirt)

D. Pink (salmon)
1. *Vibrio extorquens*
2. *Rhodococcus equi*
3. *Serratia* (some)
4. *Methylobacterium* spp.

E. Brown
1. *Bordetella pertussis*
2. *Alteromonas putrefaciens*

F. Blue-green
Pseudomonas aeruginosa (good for final identification)

G. Yellow-green
1. *Pseudomonas aeruginosa*
2. *Pseudomonas fluorescens*
3. *Pseudomonas putida*

Selected Diseases and Etiologic Agents Commonly Considered

CDC Reportable to the CDC. Individual states may have other reportable diseases not required by the CDC or other states.

Information in the table is taken from references 39 and 61; the *Manual of Clinical Microbiology*, 8th and 9th ed.; *Bailey & Scott's Diagnostic Microbiology*, 10th ed.; and the journal *Clinical Infectious Diseases*.

This table is not a complete listing of reportable diseases.

Diagnosis	Possible etiologic agent or isolates
Abscess, hepatic	Enterics, *Bacteroides*, enterococci, *Entamoeba histolytica*, *Yersinia enterocolitica*
Abscess, pancreatic	Enterics, enterococci, *Staphylococcus aureus*, coagulase-negative staphylococci, anaerobes, *Candida*
Abscess, perinephric	*S. aureus* (associated with staphylococcal bacteremia), enterics (associated with pyelonephritis)
Abscess, perirectal	Enterics, *Pseudomonas aeruginosa*, *Bacteroides*, *Enterococcus*
Abscess, pulmonary	See Pneumonia: aspiration
Abscess, splenic	*S. aureus*, streptococci, *Candida*
Abscess, tubo-ovarian	See Pelvic inflammatory disease
AIDS, pneumonia-like symptoms CDC	HIV; consider *Pneumocystis*, *Mycobacterium tuberculosis*, fungi, and any other organism
Amnionitis	See Endometritis
Anisakiasis	*Anisakis simplex* and *Pseudoterranova decipiens*
Anthrax CDC	*Bacillus anthracis*
Antibiotic rashes	Penicillins, cephalosporins, and sulfonamides; less commonly erythromycin, chloramphenicol, clindamycin, tetracyclines, and quinolones

Diagnosis	Possible etiologic agent or isolates
Arthritis, septic	Adults: *Neisseria gonorrhoeae*, *S. aureus*, streptococci, gram-negative rods rarely Infants and children: *S. aureus*, enterics, group B *Streptococcus*
Babesiosis	*Babesia microti*
Bacillary angiomatosis	*Bartonella henselae* and *B. quintana*
Balanitis	*Candida* (40%), group B *Streptococcus*, *Gardnerella*
Bilharziasis	*Schistosoma mansoni*, *S. japonicum*, *S. haematobium*
Bite, cat	*Pasteurella multocida*, *S. aureus*
Bite, dog	*P. multocida*, *S. aureus*, *Bacteroides*, *Fusobacterium*, EF-4, *Capnocytophaga*
Bite, human	Viridans group streptococci (100%), *S. epidermidis* (53%), *Corynebacterium* (41%), *S. aureus* (29%), *Eikenella* (15%), *Bacteroides* (82%)
Bite, pig	Polymicrobic; gram-positive cocci, gram-negative rods, anaerobes, *Pasteurella* spp.
Bite, prairie dog	Monkeypox virus
Bite, rat	*Spirillum minus*, *Streptobacillus moniliformis*
Blackwater fever	*Plasmodium falciparum* (kidney damage)
Bladder worm	*Taenia* cysticercus larvae
Boils	*S. aureus*
Bone: osteomyelitis (Getting a culture is critical. Ask for blood culture also. Sinus tract culture does not predict etiology of bone infection.)	*S. aureus*, gram-negative rods, and group B *Streptococcus* in newborns; group A *Streptococcus* and rarely gram-negative rods in infants older than 4 mo; enterics and *P. aeruginosa* in chronic cases
Botulism CDC	*Clostridium botulinum* toxin
Boutonneuse fever	*Rickettsia africae*
Brain abscess	*Streptococcus* spp. (60–70%), *Bacteroides* spp. (20–40%), enterics (25–33%), *S. aureus* (10–15%) (54a); if HIV positive, consider *Toxoplasma*
Brainerd diarrhea	Unknown etiology
Breast: mastitis	*S. aureus*, group A or B *Streptococcus*, enterics, *Bacteroides*, maybe *Corynebacterium*
Brill-Zinsser disease	See Typhus
Bronchiolitis	Respiratory syncytial virus (RSV) (50%), parainfluenza virus (25%), other viruses
Bronchitis	Adenovirus (in children <2 yr old), RSV, parainfluenza virus 3 (in children 2–5 yr old), viruses, *Mycoplasma pneumoniae* (5%), *Chlamydia pneumoniae* (5%) in adolescents and adults
Brucellosis CDC	*Brucella* spp. (*B. abortus*, *B. suis*, *B. melitensis*, *B. canis*)
Burn wounds	Group A *Streptococcus*, *Enterobacter*, *S. aureus*, *S. epidermidis*, *P. aeruginosa*; fungi and herpesviruses are rare causes
Candidiasis	*C. albicans* (80–90%), *C. glabrata*, *C. tropicalis*
Cat scratch disease	*Bartonella henselae*, *B. quintana*

Diagnosis	Possible etiologic agent or isolates
Cavitary pulmonary disease	*M. tuberculosis*, *Nocardia*, *Histoplasma*, *Blastomyces*, *Coccidioides*, *Aspergillus*, *Cryptococcus neoformans*
Cellulitis	*S. aureus*; group A *Streptococcus*; group B, C, and G *Streptococcus*; *Haemophilus influenzae* (periorbital)
Cercarial dermatitis (swimmer's itch)	Exposure to schistosome cercaria
Cervicitis, mucopurulent	*N. gonorrhoeae*, *Chlamydia trachomatis*
Chagas' disease	*Trypanosoma cruzi*
Chancroid	*Haemophilus ducreyi*
Chicken pox	Varicella-zoster virus (a DNA-containing herpesvirus)
Cholera	*Vibrio cholerae*
CMV	Cytomegalovirus (of the herpes group)
Coccidioidomycosis	*Coccidioides immitis*
Colorado tick fever	Caused by a coltivirus in the family *Reoviridae*
Common cold	Usually rhinoviruses (100+ serotypes); also *Mycoplasma pneumoniae*, *Chlamydia pneumoniae*
Crabs	See Pubic lice
Creeping eruption	*Ancylostoma braziliense* filariform larvae
Crohn's disease	Unknown
Croup (laryngotracheitis)	Parainfluenza virus, RSV, influenza viruses
Cryptosporidiosis	*Cryptosporidium parvum*
Cyclosporiasis	*Cyclospora*
Cysticercosis	*Taenia solium*
Dandruff: seborrheic dermatitis	*Malassezia*
Delhi boil	*Leishmania tropica*
Dental caries	*Streptococcus mutans*
Diphtheria	*Corynebacterium diphtheriae* (toxigenic)
Dumdum fever	Same as kala-azar
Ear, otitis externa (swimmer's ear)	*Pseudomonas*; enterics
Ear, otitis media (25% of the time, no etiology is determined)	

	% of isolates		
Pathogen	Neonates	Children	Adults
Streptococcus pneumoniae	20	35	21
Haemophilus influenzae	10	23	26
Moraxella catarrhalis	5	14	3
Streptococcus pyogenes		3	3
Staphylococcus aureus	17	2	3
Coagulase-negative *Staphylococcus* spp.	22		
Other bacteria	3	32	26
Viruses		16	

Diagnosis	Possible etiologic agent or isolates
Ehrlichiosis CDC	Monocytic: *E. chaffeensis*; granulocytic: *Anaplasma* (*Ehrlichia*) *phagocytophilus*
Elephantiasis	*Brugia malayi*, *Wuchereria bancrofti*
Empyema	*S. aureus*, *S. pneumoniae*, group A *Streptococcus*, *H. influenzae*, "*Streptococcus milleri*," anaerobes
Encephalitis	Arbovirus CDC, herpesvirus, West Nile virus, rabies virus (rare)
Endocarditis, native valve	Viridans group streptococci (30–40%), other streptococci (15–25%), enterococci (5–18%), *Staphylococcus* (20–35%); *Streptococcus bovis* suggests serious bowel pathology (cancer)
Endometritis	*Bacteroides*, *Prevotella bivius*, group A and B *Streptococcus*, enterics, *Chlamydia trachomatis*
Enteric fevers (typhoid and paratyphoid)	*Salmonella enterica* serovars Typhi and Paratyphi A and B
Epidimymo-orchitis	*N. gonorrhoeae* or *C. trachomatis* (patients under 35 yr old), enterics (patients over 35 yr old)
Epiglottitis	Group A *Streptococcus*, *S. aureus*, *H. influenzae* (rare)
Erysipelas	*S. pyogenes*
Erythema multiforme	Herpes simplex virus type 1, *Mycoplasma*, group A *Streptococcus*
Erythema nodosum	*S. pyogenes*; multiple others, e.g., primary tuberculosis, *Yersinia*, *Campylobacter*
Erythrasma	*Corynebacterium minutissimum*
Escherichia coli disease	Enterohemorrhagic *E. coli* (EHEC); EHEC O157:H7; EHEC Shiga toxin positive, serogroup non-O157 CDC; EHEC Shiga toxin positive, not serogrouped CDC
Eye, blepharitis	*S. aureus*; coagulase-negative *Staphylococcus*
Eye, conjunctivitis	*S. aureus*, *S. pneumoniae*, *H. influenzae* (pinkeye) Viral pinkeye: adenovirus type 3 or 7 (children); adenovirus type 8, 11, or 19 (adults) Newborns: think chemical cause; *N. gonorrhoeae*, *Chlamydia trachomatis*, herpesviruses Trachoma: *C. trachomatis*
Eye, endophthalmitis (need aspirate of vitreous humor for culture)	*S. epidermidis* (60%); *S. aureus* (5%), enterococci (5%), *Streptococcus* (5%), gram-negative rods (6%)
Fifth disease (erythema infectiosum)	Human parvovirus B19
Folliculitis	*S. aureus*, *Candida*, *P. aeruginosa*, *Malassezia*, many others; *P. aeruginosa* (whirlpool associated)

<table>
<tr><th>Diagnosis</th><th>Possible etiologic agent or isolates</th></tr>
<tr><td>Food poisoning (see 2003 Red Book [American Academy of Pediatrics]); disease due to toxins may not reveal the cultivable agent; CDC estimates 76,000,000 cases/yr (2 cases/s), with 325,000 hospitalizations and 5,000 deaths/yr</td><td>
<table>
<tr><th>Incubation period</th><th>Cause</th><th>Common vehicles</th></tr>
<tr><td>0–2 h</td><td>Mushroom toxin (early onset)</td><td>Mushrooms</td></tr>
<tr><td>0–6 h</td><td>Fish toxins</td><td>Puffer fish, shellfish, scombroid fish</td></tr>
<tr><td><1–6 h</td><td>S. aureus (toxin)</td><td>Ham, poultry, cream-filled pastry, egg and potato salad</td></tr>
<tr><td></td><td>B. cereus (emetic toxin)</td><td>Fried rice, pork</td></tr>
<tr><td>6–24 h</td><td>B. cereus (enterotoxins)</td><td>Beef, pork, vanilla sauce, chicken</td></tr>
<tr><td></td><td>C. perfringens (toxin)</td><td>Beef, poultry, gravy</td></tr>
<tr><td>16–72 h</td><td>Caliciviruses (Norwalk virus)</td><td>Shellfish, salads, ice</td></tr>
<tr><td></td><td>E. coli</td><td>Fruit, vegetables</td></tr>
<tr><td></td><td>V. cholerae</td><td>Shellfish</td></tr>
<tr><td>1–3 days</td><td>Rotavirus</td><td>Salads, fruits</td></tr>
<tr><td>16–72 h</td><td>Shigella</td><td>Egg salad, vegetables</td></tr>
<tr><td></td><td>Salmonella</td><td>Poultry, eggs, pork, dairy products</td></tr>
<tr><td></td><td>Campylobacter jejuni</td><td>Poultry, raw milk</td></tr>
<tr><td></td><td>Y. enterocolitica</td><td>Chitterlings, tofu, raw milk</td></tr>
<tr><td></td><td>V. parahaemolyticus</td><td>Fish, shellfish</td></tr>
<tr><td>12–48 h</td><td>C. botulinum</td><td>Canned vegetables, fruits, fish</td></tr>
<tr><td>72–120 h</td><td>E. coli (Shiga toxin)</td><td>Beef, raw milk, salami, dressings</td></tr>
<tr><td>1–14 days</td><td>Cyclospora sp.</td><td>Raspberries, vegetables, water</td></tr>
<tr><td></td><td>Cryptosporidium</td><td>Vegetables, fruit, water</td></tr>
<tr><td>1–4 wk</td><td>Giardia lamblia</td><td>Water, food</td></tr>
</table>
</td></tr>
<tr><td>Furunculosis</td><td>See Boils</td></tr>
<tr><td>Gallbladder infection (cholecystitis, etc.)</td><td>Enterics (68%), Enterococcus (14%), anaerobes (17%)</td></tr>
<tr><td>Gangrene, gas</td><td>Clostridium perfringens, other Clostridium spp.</td></tr>
<tr><td>Gastroenteritis, severe diarrhea (C. difficile cause must be toxin positive)</td><td>Salmonella, Shigella, Campylobacter, E. coli O157 (1–3%); culture negative?: Norwalk virus or rotavirus (rare)</td></tr>
<tr><td>Giardiasis →CDC</td><td>Giardia lamblia</td></tr>
<tr><td>Gonorrhea →CDC</td><td>Neisseria gonorrhoeae</td></tr>
<tr><td>Granuloma inguinale</td><td>Calymmatobacterium granulomatis</td></tr>
<tr><td>Hand-foot-and-mouth disease</td><td>Coxsackievirus A16 (occasionally A5 or A10)</td></tr>
<tr><td>Hemolytic-uremic syndrome</td><td>Hantavirus (also hantavirus pulmonary syndrome)</td></tr>
<tr><td>Hepatitis →CDC</td><td>Hepatitis A, B, C, D, E, and G viruses</td></tr>
<tr><td>Herpangina</td><td>Coxsackieviruses A1–A6, A8, A10</td></tr>
<tr><td>Herpetic whitlow</td><td>Herpes simplex virus on finger of health care worker, usually</td></tr>
<tr><td>Impetigo</td><td>Group A Streptococcus (contagiosa); S. aureus (bullous)</td></tr>
<tr><td>Infantile gastroenteritis</td><td>Rotavirus (30%), other astroviruses and caliciviruses, E. coli O157, Salmonella, Shigella, Campylobacter, Cryptosporidium; 33% do not show etiology</td></tr>
<tr><td>Kala-azar</td><td>Leishmania donovani</td></tr>
</table>

Diagnosis	Possible etiologic agent or isolates
Kawasaki syndrome	Unknown
Legionnaires' disease CDC	*Legionella* spp. (several)
Leprosy (Hansen's disease) CDC	*Mycobacterium leprae*
Leptospirosis	*Leptospira icterohaemorrhagiae*
Listeriosis CDC	*Listeria monocytogenes*
Ludwig's angina	Oral streptococci in submandibular space with or without *S. pyogenes*
Lyell's syndrome	See Scalded skin syndrome and Ritter's disease
Lyme disease CDC	*Borrelia burgdorferi*
Lymphogranuloma venereum	*Chlamydia trachomatis*
Malaria CDC	*Plasmodium* spp.
Measles CDC	Measles virus (single-serotype paramyxovirus)
Meningitis (aseptic): always perform STAT Gram stain to guide suspicion and therapy	Enterovirus, HSV-2, lymphochoriomeningitis virus, HIV, some drug reactions
Meningitis (bacterial): always perform STAT Gram stain to guide suspicion and therapy	<1 mo old: group B *Streptococcus*, *E. coli*, *Listeria*, gram-negative rods 1 mo–50 yr old: *S. pneumoniae*, *N. meningitidis* CDC >50 yr old: *S. pneumoniae*, *Listeria*, gram-negative rods
Mononucleosis	Epstein-Barr virus (EBV) (a herpesvirus)
Mumps CDC	Mumps virus (single-serotype paramyxovirus)
Necrotizing fasciitis ("flesh-eating bacteria")	Group A, C, and G *Streptococcus*, *Clostridium* spp., *S. aureus*
Orf	Paravaccinia virus (ovoid)
Oriental sore	See Delhi boil
Ornithosis	See Psittacosis
Osteomyelitis	*S. aureus* (up to 80%), *S. pyogenes*, *H. influenzae*, enterics less common
Pelvic inflammatory disease (PID)	*N. gonorrhoeae*, *Chlamydia*, *Bacteroides*, enterics, *Streptococcus*
Pericarditis	*S. aureus*, *S. pneumoniae*, group A *Streptococcus*, enterics
Peritonitis	Enterics (63%), *S. pneumoniae* (15%), enterococci (6–10%), anaerobes (rare) Peritoneal dialysis: *S. aureus*, *S. epidermidis*, *P. aeruginosa*, gram-negative rods
Pertussis CDC (can be a bronchitis)	*Bordetella pertussis*, rarely *B. parapertussis*
Pharyngitis	Viruses are the most common cause; group A, C, and G *Streptococcus* (A is only 10% in adults); consider mononucleosis; *C. diphtheriae*; *Arcanobacterium haemolyticum*; *Mycoplasma pneumoniae*
Plague CDC	*Yersinia pestis*
Pneumonia: aspiration	*Bacteroides*, *Peptostreptococcus*, *Fusobacterium*, *Streptococcus milleri* group, *Nocardia* (in patients taking steroids)

Diagnosis	Possible etiologic agent or isolates
Pneumonia: community and hospital acquired (CDC estimates 10,000,000 patient visits/yr with community-acquired pneumonia, i.e., >27,000/day, with 123 deaths/day)	<1 mo: CMV, rubella virus, herpesviruses, group B *Streptococcus*, *Listeria*, enterics, *S. aureus*, *P. aeruginosa* 1–3 mo: *C. trachomatis*, RSV, parainfluenza virus type 3, *Bordetella*, *S. pneumoniae* →CDC 4 mo–5 yr: RSV, other respiratory viruses, *S. pneumoniae*, *H. influenzae*, *Mycoplasma* 5–15 yr: *Mycoplasma*, *Chlamydophila pneumoniae*, *S. pneumoniae*, *M. tuberculosis*, respiratory viruses Adults: *M. pneumoniae*, *S. pneumoniae*, viruses, *M. catarrhalis*, *Legionella*, *S. aureus*
Pneumonia: interstitial (viral)	Adenovirus, hantavirus, coronavirus, influenza virus, metapneumovirus, parainfluenza virus, RSV
Polio →CDC	Poliovirus
Prion diseases	
Creutzfeldt-Jakob disease (CJD)	Prion likely
Variant CJD	Prion likely
Kuru	Prion likely
Fatal familial insomnia	Prion likely
Proctitis	See Urethritis
Prostatitis, acute	*N. gonorrhoeae* or *C. trachomatis* (patients <35 yr old), enterics (patients >35 yr old)
Prostatitis, chronic	Enterics (80%), *Enterococcus* (15%), *P. aeruginosa*
Pseudomembranous colitis	*Clostridium difficile* toxin
Pubic lice	*Phthirus pubis* and *Sarcoptes scabiei*
Pyelonephritis	Enterics (*E. coli*), enterococci
Pyoderma	*S. pyogenes* type 49
Pyomyositis	*S. aureus*, group A *Streptococcus*, rare gram-negative rods
Q fever →CDC	*Coxiella burnetii*
Rabies →CDC	Rabies virus (mostly from raccoons, not dogs, in United States)
Reiter's syndrome (urethritis, conjunctivitis, arthritis)	Occurs after infection with *C. trachomatis*, *C. jejuni*, *Y. enterocolitica*, *Salmonella*, *Shigella*; may also be poststreptococcal pharyngitis
Relapsing fever	*Borrelia recurrentis* and other *Borrelia* spp.
Rheumatic fever	Post-group A *Streptococcus* infection
Ritter's disease	*S. aureus* toxin as scalded skin syndrome
River blindness	*Onchocerca volvulus*
Rocky mountain spotted fever →CDC	*Rickettsia rickettsii*
Rubella →CDC	Rubella virus (single-serotype togavirus)
Salmonellosis →CDC	*Salmonella* spp.
Salpingitis	See Pelvic inflammatory disease
SARS (severe acute respiratory syndrome)	Caused by a coronavirus
Scabies	See Pubic lice

Diagnosis	Possible etiologic agent or isolates
Scalded skin syndrome (also called Ritter von Ritterschein disease in newborns and Ritter disease)	*S. aureus* that produces the dermolytic exotoxin
Scarlet fever	*S. pyogenes*
Sepsis	Neonates: group B *Streptococcus*, *E. coli*, *Klebsiella*, *Enterobacter* Children: *S. pneumoniae*, *N. meningitidis*, *S. aureus* Adults: Gram-negative rods, *S. aureus*, *Streptococcus*, others
Septic shock	Gram-negative rods or gram-positive cocci
Shigellosis CDC	*Shigella* spp.
Shingles	Varicella-zoster virus (herpes zoster—latent chicken pox)
Sinusitis	Acute: *S. pneumoniae* and *H. influenzae* (75%), *M. catarrhalis* (2%); group A *Streptococcus* (2%), anaerobes (6%), viruses (15%); *S. aureus* (4%) Chronic: *Prevotella*, anaerobic streptococci, *Fusobacterium*, *Streptococcus*, *Haemophilus*, *P. aeruginosa*, *Moraxella* sp.; fungi in immunocompromised patients
Slapped cheek disease	See Fifth disease
Sleeping sickness	*Trypanosoma brucei gambiense*, *T. brucei rhodesiense*
Streptococcus, "flesh eating" CDC	*Streptococcus pyogenes* (invasive)
Syphilis CDC	*Treponema pallidum*
Tetanus CDC	*Clostridium tetani*
Thrombophlebitis	*Streptococcus*, *Bacteroides*, enterics
Thrombosis	*S. aureus*, group A *Streptococcus*, *H. influenzae*, *Aspergillus*, *Mucor*, *Rhizopus*
Toxic shock syndrome CDC	*S. aureus* that produces the toxin; group A, B, C, and G *Streptococcus*
Toxoplasmosis	*Toxoplasma gondii* (a protozoan)
Trench fever	*Bartonella quintana*
Trichomoniasis	*Trichomonas vaginalis*
Tuberculosis CDC	*Mycobacterium tuberculosis*
Tularemia CDC	*Francisella tularensis*
Typhoid fever CDC	*Salmonella typhi*
Typhus	*Rickettsia prowazekii* (louse borne), *Rickettsia typhi* (murine), *Orientia tsutsugamushi* (scrub typhus)
Ulcer, decubitus (culture tissue samples, not swabs)	Polymicrobic; beta-hemolytic *Streptococcus*, enterococci, anaerobic *Streptococcus*, enterics, *Pseudomonas*, *S. aureus*
Ulcer, duodenal or gastric	*Helicobacter pylori*
Urethritis	*N. gonorrhoeae* (50% also have concomitant *C. trachomatis* infection)
Urethritis, nongonococcal	*Chlamydia* (50%), *Mycoplasma hominis*, *Ureaplasma*, *Trichomonas*, *Mycoplasma genitalium*
Urinary tract infection (uncomplicated)	Enterics (*E. coli*), *Staphylococcus saprophyticus*, enterococci
Vaginosis, bacterial	Polymicrobic; diagnose by Gram stain, not culture
Vincent's angina	Anaerobes, spirochetes
Warts, genital	Papillomavirus
Whipple's disease	*Tropheryma whipplei*
Wounds	Polymicrobic; *S. aureus*, group A *Streptococcus*, enterics, *Clostridium*

The Top 10 Notifiable Infectious Diseases in the United States, According to the *Morbidity and Mortality Weekly Report*

Disease	No. of cases/100,000 population in 2004
1. Chlamydia (sexually transmitted)	319.6
2. Gonorrhea	113.5
3. AIDS	15.2
4. Salmonellosis	14.5
5. Syphilis (all stages)	11.5
6. Varicella (chicken pox)	18.4
7. Pertussis	8.9
8. Giardiasis	8.3
9. Lyme disease	6.8
10. Shigellosis	5.0

Can I Do a Disk Susceptibility Test on That Isolate? Organisms That Have Specific Interpretive Criteria Available through CLSI Standards (21)[a]

Organism(s)[b]	Medium for testing
Acinetobacter spp.	Routine MH agar
Burkholderia cepacia	Routine MH agar
Enterobacteriaceae	Routine MH agar
Enterococcus spp.	Routine MH agar
Haemophilus influenzae, H. parainfluenzae	HTM in CO_2
Neisseria gonorrhoeae	GC agar base + supplement in CO_2
Neisseria meningitidis	MH + 5% sheep blood in CO_2
Pseudomonas aeruginosa	Routine MH agar
Staphylococcus aureus, S. lugdunensis, CNS for MecA	Routine MH agar + cefoxitin disk
Staphylococcus spp.	Routine MH agar
Stenotrophomonas maltophilia	Routine MH agar
Streptococcus pneumoniae	MH + 5% sheep blood in CO_2
Streptococcus spp. (not *S. pneumoniae*)	MH + 5% sheep blood in CO_2
Vibrio cholerae	Routine MH agar

[a]MH, Mueller-Hinton agar supplemented with Ca^{2+} and Mg^{2+} incubated in ambient air unless otherwise noted; HTM, *Haemophilus* test medium; GC, gonococcus; CNS, coagulase-negative staphylococci.

[b]If the species of bacteria to be tested does not appear on this list, the disk test cannot be used for routine antimicrobial susceptibility testing because there are no interpretive criteria yet available for that organism.

Can I Do an MIC Susceptibility Test on That Isolate? Organisms That Have Specific Interpretive Criteria Available through CLSI Standards (21)

Organism(s)[a]	Medium for testing[b]
Acinetobacter spp.	CAMHB
Bioterrorism agents: *Bacillus anthracis, Yersinia pestis, Burkholderia mallei, B. pseudomallei, Francisella tularensis, Brucella* spp.	Refer to LRN laboratory for testing: CLSI recommends CAMHB, CAMHB + supplements, or brucella broth, depending on the isolate
Burkholderia cepacia	CAMHB
Enterobacteriaceae	CAMHB
Enterococcus spp.	CAMHB
Haemophilus influenzae, H. parainfluenzae	HTM broth
Helicobacter pylori	Agar dilution in MH agar + aged sheep blood
Neisseria gonorrhoeae	Agar dilution with GC base + supplement in CO_2
Neisseria meningitidis	CAMHB + 5% lysed horse blood in CO_2
Pseudomonas aeruginosa; other *Pseudomonas* spp.; other nonfastidious, nonfermentative gram-negative rods	CAMHB
Staphylococcus spp.	CAMHB (perhaps supplemented with 2% NaCl)
Stenotrophomonas maltophilia	CAMHB
Streptococcus pneumoniae	CAMHB + 5% lysed horse blood in air
Streptococcus spp. (not *S. pneumoniae*)	CAMHB + 5% lysed horse blood
Vibrio cholerae	CAMHB

[a]If the species to be tested is not listed in this table, it does not have interpretive criteria available from CLSI. Other organisms may be tested by the MIC procedure, but only the MIC value may be reported, not "susceptible," "intermediate," or "resistant."

[b]CAMHB, cation-supplemented Mueller-Hinton broth incubated in ambient air unless otherwise noted; HTM, *Haemophilus* test medium; GC, gonococcus.

SECTION III
Communicating the Results

The therapeutic information in the following chart is not intended to guide therapy by a clinician but rather to inform laboratorians of the options available. 1st Rx, drug of choice; 2nd Rx, secondary drug of choice; AFB, acid-fast bacilli; anaBA, anaerobic blood agar; AST, antimicrobial susceptibility test; BA, blood agar; CDC, Centers for Disease Control and Prevention; f., formerly called; LAP, leucine aminopeptidase test; LKV, laked blood with kanamycin and vancomycin agar for anaerobes; MIC, minimum inhibitory concentration test (by automated instrument); PYR, pyrrolidonyl arylamidase; S, I, and R, susceptible, intermediate, and resistant, respectively; K/B, Kirby/Bauer; BBE, *Bacteroides* bile esculin; Ig, immunoglobulin; SXT, trimethoprim-sulfamethoxazole; ID, identification; CLSI, Clinical and Laboratory Standards Institute (formerly NCCLS); ELISA, enzyme-linked immunosorbent assay; GI, gastrointestinal; ESBLs, extended-spectrum beta-lactamases; IIF, indirect immunofluorescence; CF, complement fixation; SPS, sodium polyanethol sulfonate; DFA, direct fluorescent antibody; IFA, indirect fluorescent antibody; EIA, enzyme immunoassay; AMP, ampicillin; HPS, hantavirus pulmonary syndrome; BE, bile esculin; HAV, hepatitis A virus; ssRNA, single-stranded RNA; TB, tuberculosis; TM, Thayer-Martin; PEN, penicillin; RMSF, Rocky mountain spotted fever; MRSA, methicillin-resistant *S. aureus*; V, variable; WHO, World Health Organization.

☣ Do not attempt to identify these isolates. These organisms are on the HHS or overlap select agent or toxin list and must be sent to a Laboratory Response Network (LRN) laboratory for identification, secured in the laboratory while at the reference lab, and destroyed or transferred to a registered laboratory after the identification has been confirmed.

NCCLS proposed standard M38-P is for testing filamentous fungi. Most clinical microbiology laboratories will not provide this service due to lack of resources and training, but reference laboratories should provide susceptibility testing.

The website from which updated information, particularly regarding viruses, was obtained was the Centers for Disease Control and Prevention site at www.cdc.gov. Information on yeasts and fungi was taken from the Doctor Fungus website at www.doctorfungus.com, and the descriptions and susceptibility data were used with permission. Similar formats are available elsewhere (45a).

Antimicrobial information is from references 2, 23, and 39. It is for lab information only. Therapeutic decisions must be made by the physician. Some information on the extent of identification and the comments are from references 23, 37, 44, 48, and 63a.

Organism	Antimicrobic information	Extent of identification and comments
Abiotrophia spp. (f. nutritionally deficient streptococcus; see also *Granulicatella*) One species: *A. defectiva* (63).	Do not do AST. If clinically necessary, refer. Susceptible to clindamycin, rifampin, levofloxacin, ofloxacin, and quinupristin-dalfopristin (72).	Normal flora of oral cavity but can be found in endocarditis. Requires supplement for growth: 1. Streak a lawn of the isolate (usually from blood bottle) and do a single streak of *S. aureus* ATCC 25923. Incubate at 35°C in CO_2 and look for satelliting, or 2. Use media supplemented with pyridoxal (final concentration of 0.001%) or use a Remel pyridoxal disk.
Absidia (f. *Mucor corymbifer*) One of the Zygomycetes. Twenty-one species with *A. corymbifera* the most common.	Limited data on susceptibility. Amphotericin B is active against this organism, but azoles are not.	Filamentous fungus, ubiquitous, common environmental contaminant. May cause food spoilage. Rare as a cause of human disease.
Achromobacter (f. Vd-1,2) Name has changed; now *Ochrobactrum anthropi.* Also see *Alcaligenes.*	Do not test. Refer. You can try a conventional MIC and report value only, not S-I-R. **1st Rx:** imipenem, ceftazidime, meropenem **2nd Rx:** SXT, fluoroquinolone, ticarcillin/clavulanate	
Acidovorax spp. Recently described genus.	No interpretive guidelines available. Do *not* do disk test with these isolates. Use MIC only and use *P. aeruginosa* interpretive standards (40). Therapy depends on susceptibility test.	Gram-negative rods that may be slightly curved. Three species, all rare in humans and questionably pathogenic. Common in environment (water, soil, plants) and aerobic.
***Acinetobacter baumannii* complex** (f. *Acinetobacter calcoaceticus* subsp. *anitratus* or *A. nitratus*; name changed) Use the name currently on the database of your ID instrument.	Use K/B, MIC, or Etest. **1st Rx:** imipenem or meropenem (fluoroquinolone + amikacin) **2nd Rx:** ampicillin/sulbactam 5% resistant to imipenem. Often resistant to penicillin, ampicillin, chloramphenicol. Combination Rx with beta-lactam and aminoglycoside may be needed for serious cases. Can do disk, MIC, and Etest and interpret with *Pseudomonas* breakpoints. Always confirm if resistant to colistin.	~50% from urinary tract infections; also ear, eye, nose, throat. Normal on skin and in feces. This organism is of nosocomial importance. Oxidase negative (good clue).
Acinetobacter lwoffii		Inert, oxidase negative. Often resistant to penicillin; sensitive to most other antimicrobials.
Acremonium (f. *Cephalosporium*) Three species of importance: *A. falciforme*, *A. kiliense*, and *A. recifei.*	Limited data but amphotericin B is active. May also respond to azoles +/– amphotericin B.	Filamentous fungus from plants and soils. Rapid grower, maturing by 5 days. May or may not be implicated infection since it can be a contaminant. May be confused with *Fusarium* without macroconidia.

Actinobacillus actinomycetemcomitans	Information for all five species listed here: no CLSI test method exists. Test should be referred if requested. Often resistant to penicillin. Not usually tested but MIC or Etest may be used to report only MIC value, not S-I-R.	Normal oral flora. May be associated with *Actinomyces israelii.* Needs serum and carbon dioxide for best growth. Note "star" colony. May be granular at bottom/sides of broth tube. Rough, "sticky" colony on BA, as if it were glued onto the plate.
Actinobacillus equuli		From donkey bites and pigs. Rare in humans but found in joint fluid, wounds. Sticky colony whose character is not lost on subculture. PEN resistance has been reported.
Actinobacillus lignieresii		Obtained from horse bites and monkeys. Rare in humans. Sticky colony lost on subculture. Tiny cells on BA, long cells on glucose-containing media.
Actinobacillus suis		Similar biochemically to *A. equuli.* Colony not as sticky as *A. equuli* but gets stickier by 72 h. This is the only esculin-positive *Actinobacillus* species.
Actinobacillus ureae (f. *Pasteurella ureae*)		Rare in humans but most from UTIs. Bizarre morphology, wide cells with vacuoles. Actinobacilli are genetic relatives of *Pasteurella.* Actinobacilli grow on MacConkey agar; common *Pasteurella* spp. do not.
Actinomadura An aerobic actinomycete. Genus has 27 species, including 3 that infect humans: *A. madurae*, *A. pelletieri*, and *A. dassonvillei.*	Combination therapy often preferred: streptomycin and dapsone for *A. madurae*, streptomycin and SXT for *A. pelletieri.*	A filamentous soil bacterium. Causes mycetoma (maduramycosis or madura foot). Commonly produces granules containing branched filaments. Waxy-like colony or orange, red, pink, yellow, white, tan. Acid-fast stain results: *Actinomadura* (negative); *Nocardiopsis* (negative), *Streptomyces* (most are negative); *Nocardia* (positive).
Actinomadura madurae	No CLSI criteria. Do not test. Refer.	Aerobic actinomycete. Gram positive, nonfragmenting with partial branching and sparse aerial hyphae that each carry up to 15 arthrospores (76).
Actinomyces israelii	Do not test. Refer. No CLSI interpretive criteria exist. **1st Rx:** penicillins, ampicillin or imipenem **2nd Rx:** doxycycline or erythromycin or ceftriaxone Resistant to metronidazole. Not routinely tested, but CLSI does have an anaerobic procedure (39).	Anaerobic but may grow in CO_2. Catalase-negative, gram-positive rods. Not acid-fast (*Nocardia* is partially acid-fast). Can use RapID ANA II.
Actinomyces naeslundii		Same comment and drugs as *Actinomyces israelii.* Can use RapID ANA II.
Adenovirus According to the CDC, there are 49 immunologically distinct types (six subgenera: A–F) that can cause human infections. Acute respiratory disease is most often associated with adenoviruses 4 and 7 in the United States. Enteric adenoviruses 40 and 41 cause gastroenteritis, usually in children.	There is no virus-specific therapy available. Most infections are mild and require no therapy or only symptomatic treatment. Serious illness is managed by treating symptoms and complications of the infection. Vaccines for adenovirus serotypes 4 and 7 have been available only for preventing acute respiratory disease among military recruits.	Usually causes respiratory illness; various serotypes may also cause gastroenteritis, conjunctivitis, cystitis, and rash illness. All are transmitted by direct contact, fecal-oral transmission, and, occasionally, waterborne transmission. Adenovirus 7 acquired by inhalation is associated with severe lower respiratory tract disease, whereas oral transmission of the virus is often innocuous. **Serology:** Can order complement fixation and ELISA for genus-specific antibody, serum neutralization and hemagglutination inhibition for type-specific antibody, and in situ hybridization and immunofluorescence for antigen detection.

<table>
<tr><th>Organism</th><th>Antimicrobic information</th><th>Extent of identification and comments</th></tr>
<tr><td>Aerococcus spp.
Often contaminants but may be important in endocarditis and bacteremia. A. urinae recently found in patients predisposed to UTIs.</td><td>Can do conventional MIC or use instrument but only report MIC value without interpretations. No CLSI criteria are available. Both species are susceptible to penicillin and vancomycin. Erythromycin and tetracycline may also work, but some resistance has been noted (63).</td><td>Usually PYR positive, LAP negative, bile esculin (variable), NaCl positive.
With a staphylococcus-like Gram stain, A. urinae is PYR negative and vancomycin susceptible and grows in 6.5% NaCl.
A. viridans is PYR positive and LAP negative and also grows in 6.5% NaCl.</td></tr>
<tr><td>Aeromonas caviae (1)
Nonhemolytic on BA.
A. caviae complex consists of A. caviae, A. media, and A. eucrennophila.</td><td>No specific CLSI interpretive criteria exist; however, these organisms would be covered under the Pseudomonas and other non-Enterobacteriaceae charts.
Can also do conventional or instrument MIC or Etest and report the MIC value with or without the S-I-R.</td><td>At least 10 species of Aeromonas exist.
Mostly aquatic organisms worldwide, inhabiting fresh, polluted, brackish, or chlorinated water. Disease caused by ingestion of contaminated food, skin exposure, fish fins, or hooks. Virulence role is uncertain: wounds, bacteremia, endocarditis, meningitis, pneumonia.
Most colonies are large, round, opaque, nonhemolytic.</td></tr>
<tr><td>Aeromonas hydrophila (1)
A. hydrophila complex consists of A. hydrophila, A. bestiarum, and A. salmonicida.</td><td>For GI infections, therapy usually not needed.
Bacteremia: fluoroquinolones or expanded- or broad-spectrum cephalosporin, imipenem, aztreonam.
1st Rx: fluoroquinolone
2nd Rx: SXT
Aeromonas and Plesiomonas shigelloides can produce various beta-lactamases (35).</td><td>Accuracy of most automated systems is unpredictable. Requires confirmation by conventional testing.

To separate Aeromonas from Vibrio:
<table><tr><th></th><th>Aeromonas</th><th>V. fluvialis</th></tr><tr><td>β-Glucosidase</td><td>>90%</td><td>29%</td></tr><tr><td>PYR</td><td>0%</td><td>68%</td></tr></table>
To separate Aeromonas, Plesiomonas, and Vibrio spp. (28):
<table><tr><th></th><th>Lysine</th><th>Arginine</th><th>Ornithine</th><th>0% NaCl</th></tr><tr><td>Plesiomonas</td><td>+</td><td>+</td><td>+</td><td>+</td></tr><tr><td>Aeromonas</td><td>V</td><td>−</td><td>+</td><td>+</td></tr><tr><td>Vibrio</td><td>+</td><td>+</td><td>−</td><td>V</td></tr></table></td></tr>
<tr><td>Aeromonas sobria (1)
These are actually A. veronii bv. sobria and should be reported correctly.
A. veronii bv. sobria is a symbiont in the gut of leeches.</td><td></td><td></td></tr>
<tr><td>Afipia spp.
Named for the Armed Forces Institute of Pathology, where they were first described as the agent of cat scratch disease (see Bartonella).
Genus consists of A. felis, A. broomeae, A. clevelandensis, and three unnamed species.</td><td>Refer for testing. More resistant than Bartonella spp. in vitro; A. felis is susceptible to imipemem, aminoglycoside, and rifampin. Resistant to penicillin, cephalosporin, and fluoroquinolones (76).</td><td>All are urease and oxidase positive (Bartonella are negative). Facultative intracellular pathogen, grows a little faster than Bartonella, less fastidious.
Grows best at 30°C. Colonies develop by 72 h on blood agar or buffered charcoal yeast extract. Resist serology testing for Afipia as a cause of cat scratch disease; only Bartonella will be positive.</td></tr>
</table>

Agrobacterium radiobacter (f. Vd-3 and *Agrobacterium tumefaciens*)	No CLSI interpretive criteria. Try conventional MIC or Etest but otherwise refer it for testing.	Environmental organism isolated from wounds, sputum, eye infections.
Alcaligenes faecalis (f. *Alcaligenes odorans*; CDC VI) The asaccharolytic member of this oxidase-positive, motile, nonfermenter group, along with *Achromobacter piechaudii* and *Achromobacter xylosoxidans* subsp. *denitrificans.* ***Alcaligenes xylosoxidans*** ***Alcaligenes denitrificans*** (now *Achromobacter*) The saccharolytic members of this oxidase-positive, motile, nonfermenter group now called *Achromobacter xylosoxidans* subsp. *xylosoxidans*, which contains three additional unnamed groups, B, E, and F.	No CLSI method or interpretations. May do conventional MIC and report the value only. **1st Rx:** imipenem; meropenem; antipseudomonals; penicillin **2nd Rx:** SXT Resistant to aminoglycosides and quinolones.	Taxonomy of this genus is somewhat confusing. *A. faecalis* spreads like a bacillus, smells like apples, and causes browning in blood agar.
Alishewanella fetalis (74)	No data available.	Nonmotile, nonfermentative gram-negative bacterium isolated from a human fetus in Sweden and easily misidentified as *Shewanella putrefaciens*. Its close taxonomic relationship supplies its new name.
Alternaria Contains about 50 species, but *A. alternate* is most common in humans.	Standard procedures not yet developed for testing. Caspofungin, voriconazole, amphotericin B, flucytosine active in vitro. Fluconazole may also work.	A dematiaceous fungus that is common on plants, in soil, and in indoor air. Usually a contaminant but considered opportunistic in immunocompromised patients. Greenish-black to olive-brown pigment.
Alteromonas putrefaciens Incorrect name; see *Shewanella putrefaciens*		
Amp-C beta-lactamase	An Ambler class C beta-lactamase primarily produced in *E. cloacae* and *C. freundii*, with similar enzymes in *Serratia marcescens*, *Morganella morganii*, *Providencia stuartii*, and *Providencia rettgeri*. This class of enzymes is better at degrading cephalosporins than penicillins. Causes resistance to all penicillins and cephalosporins except carbapenems. They are not inhibited by clavulanate like ESBLs are. Turn on the appropriate "flags" for MicroScan and Vitek detection. A disk test is available based on use of Tris-EDTA to make a bacterial cell permeable and release beta-lactamases into the external environment. Amp-C disks (i.e., filter paper disks containing Tris-EDTA) available from BD Diagnostic Systems, Sparks, MD (9). Other disk combinations have been reported (25).	

<table>
<tr><th>Organism</th><th>Antimicrobic information</th><th>Extent of identification and comments</th></tr>
<tr>
<td>Anaerobic bacteria (20)</td>
<td>
See Flowcharts 4 and 5 for recognizing and grouping anaerobes.
In most cases, anaerobic susceptibility need not be done. If it is specifically requested by the physician, refer to a reference laboratory.

Empiric therapy
<table>
<tr><th></th><th>1st Rx</th><th>2nd Rx</th></tr>
<tr><td>B. fragilis</td><td>Metronidazole</td><td>Clindamycin</td></tr>
<tr><td>C. difficile</td><td>Metronidazole (per os)</td><td>Vancomycin (per os)</td></tr>
<tr><td>C. perfringens</td><td>Penicillin + clindamycin</td><td>Doxycycline</td></tr>
<tr><td>C. tetani</td><td>Metronidazole, penicillin</td><td>Doxycycline</td></tr>
</table>

In vitro data indicate the following:
Prevotella: susceptible to expanded- and broad-spectrum cephalosporins, penicillins (if beta-lactamase negative), clindamycin, trovafloxacin.
Porphyromonas: same as Prevotella.
Fusobacterium: same as Prevotella.
Veillonella: susceptible to chloramphenicol, clindamycin, imipenem, meropenem, metronidazole, ticarcillin.
Always confirm if any anaerobe is resistant to metronidazole.
</td>
<td>
Gram-negative anaerobic bacteria
1. Large colonies on anaBA with corresponding gray or black colonies on BBE and regular gram-negative rods are Bacteroides fragilis group at 95%.
2. Bread crumb or opalescent colonies on anaBA that do not grow on BBE, are spot indole positive, and have thin, pointed fusiform cells are Fusobacterium nucleatum at 95%.
3. Small (<1 mm) translucent colonies on anaBA and BBE after 48 h with a black dot in the center (H_2S) and catalase positive are Bilophila wadsworthia.
4. Black-pigmented colonies or those that fluoresce red with long-wave UV on LKV with corresponding colonies on anaBA that are small coccobacilli are of a Prevotella sp. If these are spot indole positive, they are Prevotella intermedia.
5. Organisms with similar colonies on anaBA, red fluorescence with UV, and similar Gram stain morphology but no growth on LKV and are indole positive are Porphyromonas spp.
6. Flat, transparent colonies that pit the agar, are catalase negative and urea positive, and fail to grow on BBE are Bacteroides ureolyticus.
7. Small, transparent-to-opaque colonies on anaBA that fluoresce red with UV, do not grow on BBE, and are gram-negative diplococci are Veillonella spp.
Gram-positive anaerobic bacteria
1. Large irregular colonies, double zone of beta-hemolysis on anaerobic blood agar (anaBA), no growth on BBE, catalase negative, large, boxcar-shaped, blunt, gram-positive rods without spores on Gram stain are Clostridium perfringens.
C. perfringens epsilon toxin is on the select agent/toxin list. C. botulinum is on the overlap list.
2. Smoothly swarming growth on anaBA, spot indole negative, catalase negative, thin gram-positive rods with swollen subterminal spores on Gram stain is Clostridium septicum. (Associated with colon cancers.)
3. Slow swarmer on anaBA, spot indole positive, catalase negative, and gram positive with swollen terminal spores (tennis-racket shape) is Clostridium tetani (rarely seen).
4. Slowly swarming growth, serpentine-edged colonies, spot indole positive, urea positive, catalase negative, subterminal spores is Clostridium sordellii.
5. Small, enamel-white colonies on anaBA, no growth on BBE, spot indole positive, catalase positive, and pleomorphic coryneform rods are Propionibacterium acnes.
6. Thin, spore-forming gram-positive rods (spores rarely visible). Colonies on cycloserine-cefoxitin-fructose agar are large and flat. If one of these organisms has chartreuse fluorescence on anaBA and smells like a barnyard, it is Clostridium difficile.
</td>
</tr>
</table>

Anaplasma phagocytophila (f. *Ehrlichia*)	No test method available. **1st Rx:** doxycycline **2nd Rx:** tetracycline Resistant to clindamycin, SXT, imipenem, penicillin, ampicillin, and erythromycin.	Causes human granulocytic ehrlichiosis. Giemsa or Wright stain positive in 60% of patients. Transmitted by *Ixodes scapularis* (deer tick), *I. pacificus* (western black-legged tick), *I. ricinus* (rabbit tick). PCR available. EDTA blood cultured into HL-60 or THP1 cell lines will be positive in 3–30 days if inoculated prior to administration of antibiotics. Indirect fluorescent antibody (IFA) serology is available and is effective.
Antimicrobial susceptibility results that require confirmation either in-house or by a reference laboratory (51)	Any anaerobe resistant to metronidazole. *Acinetobacter* resistant to colistin. *Bacteroides* resistant to metronidazole, amoxicillin/clavulanic acid, or carbapenems. *Clostridium difficile* resistant to metronidazole or vancomycin. Coagulase-negative staphylococcus resistant to vancomycin or linezolid. *Corynebacterium jeikeium* resistant to vancomycin, teicoplanin, or linezolid. *Enterobacteriaceae* resistant to meropenem or imipenem (except with *Proteus* spp.). Enterococci resistant to both ampicillin and quinupristin-dalfopristin; linezolid, or teicoplanin, but not vancomycin. Group A, B, C, G streptococci resistant to penicillin, vancomycin, teicoplanin, or linezolid. *Haemophilus influenzae* resistant to any third-generation cephalosporin or carbapenem. *Moraxella catarrhalis* resistant to ciprofloxacin. *Neisseria gonorrhoeae* resistant to any third-generation cephalosporin. *Neisseria meningitidis* resistant to any penicillin or ciprofloxacin. *Staphylococcus aureus* resistant to vancomycin, teicoplanin, linezolid, or quinupristin-dalfopristin. *Streptococcus pneumoniae* resistant to meropenem, vancomycin, teicoplanin, or linezolid.	
Arboviruses Includes more than 150 arthropod-borne viruses. Includes hantaviruses and California encephalitis, Colorado tick fever, dengue, Ebola, Japanese encephalitis, LaCrosse, eastern equine encephalitis, Venezuelan equine encephalitis, western equine encephalitis, St. Louis encephalitis, Lassa fever, Marburg, Rift Valley fever, vesicular stomatitis, West Nile, and yellow fever viruses.	No specific therapy available.	**Serology:** IgM and IgG ELISA, IIF, hemagglutination inhibition, and CF are available for yellow fever, dengue, eastern equine encephalitis, Venezuelan equine encephalitis, and western equine encephalitis, but only IgG ELISA is available for Colorado tick fever. Serum neutralization is available for yellow fever and dengue.
Arcanobacterium haemolyticum (f. *Corynebacterium haemolyticum*) Five recognized species. *A. haemolyticum*, *A. bernardiae*, and *A. pyogenes* have been isolated from humans.	No CLSI interpretive criteria. Resist testing or refer or do MIC or Etest and report MIC data only. Generally susceptible to most drugs except SXT. **1st Rx:** erythromycin or penicillin (14, 39)	Associated with pharyngitis, abscesses, wounds, and cutaneous/rash infections. Irregular, gram-positive rods that are catalase negative and nonmotile. Looks like small streptococcal colony—negative latex (but may show weak group F+). Growth on BA better than on chocolate agar. Occurs more frequently in 10- to 22-yr-olds vs. group A streptococcus, which peaks in <10-yr-olds. In healthy throats, about 1 in 800 (4, 19).

Organism	Antimicrobic information	Extent of identification and comments
Arcobacter spp. Two of the four species have been from human infections: *A. butzleri* and *A. cryaerophilus.*	No CLSI criteria for testing.	Gram-negative, curved or helical rods. Aerotolerant, *Campylobacter*-like organisms. No antigen tests defined. Culture by growing below 35°C. No growth at 42°C; microaerophilic and can grow on selective media, e.g. Campy-CVA medium (57).
Arthrobacter spp. *A. cumminsii* (most common human isolate), *A. creatinolyticus, A. luteolus, A. albus.*	See Diphtheroids.	Usually called diphtheroid or coryneform. Normal soil habitat and may be normal in humans. Inert to sugars and does *not* smell like cheese, unlike brevibacteria.
Arthrographis Five species, with *A. kalrae* most common in humans.	No standardized tests, but publications have shown that amphotericin B, fluconazole, itraconazole, and miconazole may be effective (17, 78).	A filamentous fungus that has been associated with mycetoma, contact lens infections, sinusitis, and other problems in immunocompromised patients.
Asaia Primarily environmental. ***A. bogorensis*** Rare in humans. ***A. krungthepensis*** ***A. siamensis*** Not yet an approved name.	Submit to reference laboratory. Recent human bacteremia isolate in Finland resistant to most gram-negative antimicrobials but susceptible to netilmicin, gentamicin, and doxycycline (79).	Gram-negative, aerobic rod. Peritrichous flagella. Initially isolated from flowers of the orchid tree and of plumbago in Indonesia. Grows at pH 3.0 and at 30°C.
***Aureobacterium* spp.**	No CLSI interpretive criteria available. Send out or do conventional MIC on gram-positive panel and report MIC values only. *Alert:* Vancomycin resistance reported (58) in a case of cellulitis and fatal septicemia and in a patient with acute myelogenous leukemia with concomitant porphyria cutanea tarda.	Other catalase-positive, yellow-pigmented, irregular gram-positive rods include *Microbacterium, Oerskovia, Cellulomonas, Brevibacterium,* and *Corynebacterium aquaticum.* Catalase-positive, yellow-pigmented, irregular gram-positive rods with oxidative metabolism—from plants, milk, dairy products, soil, sewage, and insects. A diphtheroid similar to *Corynebacterium aquaticum*, except for gelatin hydrolysis, casein hydrolysis, and more rapidly appearing pigment in *Aureobacterium.*
***Bacillus* spp.** ☣ (*B. anthracis*) 9 new genera from this group (52): *Alicyclobacillus, Ammoniphilus, Amphibacillus, Gracilibacillus, Halobacillus, Salibacillus, Sulfobacillus, Thermobacillus,* and *Ureibacillus*	The resistance of *B. cereus* to most beta-lactams makes vancomycin the drug of choice. Can also use clindamycin, a fluoroquinolone, or imipenem for either *B. cereus* or *B. subtilis.* Test *B. anthracis* only with penicillin, tetracycline, and ciprofloxacin.	*Bacillus* spp. may or may not be a contaminant. Often a contaminant in blood cultures. (*If from blood and the patient is alive, it is likely not B. anthracis*, but this is not a definitive observation.) If from a sterile site, do a cefinase test: if negative, document on work card only. If positive, report "beta-lactamase positive."

are unlikely to be isolated from humans. Also contains *Paenibacillus* (27 species, f. *B. polymyxa*, *B. macerans*, *B. alvei*, and the pathogens *B. larvae* and *B. pulvifaciens*), *Aneurinibacillus*, *Virgibacillus*, and *Geobacillus* (8 thermophiles including *B. stearothermophilus*).	*B. anthracis*: **1st Rx:** ciprofloxacin or doxycycline **2nd Rx:** penicillin G or amoxicillin	Risk factors for bacteremia: vascular catheter; intravenous drug abuse; cancer, especially *B. cereus* in granulocytopenic patients with hematologic neoplasms. Catalase positive and motile by peritrichous flagella. Do not attempt workup if *B. anthracis* is suspected; ship directly to LRN reference laboratory. The edges of *B. anthracis* colonies can be lifted up like stiff egg whites. Spore formation occurs only under aerobic conditions; will not see spores in direct tissue stains.
Bartonella* spp.** (f. *Rochalimaea*) Four species associated with humans. ***B. bacilliformis Causes Oroya fever. From the Andes Mountains of South America. Has a sand fly vector. ***B. quintana*** Trench fever; global; vector is *Pediculus humanus* (body louse). ***B. henselae*** Cat scratch disease. Globally endemic. Transmitted by cats and cat fleas (76).	No test method available. Refer. Etest has been used successfully. Susceptible to many agents in vitro including beta-lactams, tetracycline, erythromycin, aminoglycoside, fluoroquinolone, vancomycin, chloramphenicol, and SXT. Resistant to nalidixic acid, and some penicillin resistance has been noted (76). **1st Rx:** erythromycin or doxycycline (bacillary angiomatosis) or azithromycin (cat scratch) **2nd Rx:** clarithromycin or ciprofloxacin	Grows on BA in air or CO_2. Human-associated strains best at 25–30°C (*B. bacilliformis*) to 35–37°C (*B. henselae*, *B. quintana*, and *B. elizabethae*). May be a mixture of dry and moist, adhering colonies. Named after A. L. Barton. Small gram-negative rods, slightly curved. Oxidase negative, aerobic, highly fastidious, intraerythrocytic. **Serology:** Skin testing is available for cat scratch disease, and IIF can detect antibodies.
***Baylisascaris* spp.** (intestinal raccoon roundworm) Rare but does cause human disease in the United States.		People become infected by accidentally ingesting infective eggs from soil, water, or things contaminated with raccoon feces. Rarely causes disease in raccoons. In humans, may migrate to internal organs.
Bergeyella zoohelcum (f. *Weeksella zoohelcum*)	See *Weeksella*.	
Bipolaris *B. spicifera*, *B. australiensis*, and *B. hawaiiensis* are the most common of several species.	Amphotericin B, ketoconazole (itraconazole and voriconazole also may be effective). Refer for susceptibility if warranted.	Dematiaceous, filamentous fungus. One of the potential causes of phaeohyphomycosis and may be superficial, cutaneous, subcutaneous, corneal, respiratory, or systemic.
Blastocystis hominis	**1st Rx:** metronidazole	Formerly considered a yeast, this is now classified as a protozoan along with other amoebae. May be found in up to 20% of healthy populations but if present in large numbers in the absence of other intestinal pathogens, this is often considered a pathogen. Controversy remains as to its pathogenicity.

<table>
<tr><th>Organism</th><th>Antimicrobic information</th><th>Extent of identification and comments</th></tr>
<tr><td>Blastomyces dermatitidis
The only species in its genus. Sexual stage is Ajellomyces dermatitidis.</td><td>No standard testing available. Submit to reference laboratory. Responds to amphotericin B, ketoconazole, and itraconazole; secondary choice is fluconazole.</td><td>A true systemic mycosis. A chronic infection often beginning as respiratory illness and then spreading to skin and other organs. To identify, lab must convert isolate from the mold at 25°C to a yeast phase at 37°C. The Mississippi, Ohio, and Missouri valleys are the geographic locations with highest incidence in the United States.
Serology: Antibodies develop, but current serology is unreliable.</td></tr>
<tr><td>Blastoschizomyces capitatus
(f. Trichosporon capitatum and Geotrichum capitatum)
The only species in its genus.</td><td>No standard testing available. Submit to reference laboratory. Fluconazole and 5-fluorocytosine may be helpful (23).</td><td>A yeast considered normal environmental flora. Rare cause of disease in immunocompromised patients. Systemic disease is very dangerous. Morphologically and phenotypically resembles Candida krusei and Trichosporon spp.</td></tr>
<tr><td>Blood cultures (general information)
Sources of bacteremia (8)
Intravascular devices: 19%
Genitourinary tract: 17%
Respiratory tract: 12%
Abscesses: 10%
Surgical site infections: 5%
Biliary tract: 5%
Other known sites: 8%
Unknown: 27%</td><td colspan="2">Invasion of blood either by drainage from a primary focus of infection via the lymphatic system to the vascular system or direct entry from needles, intravascular devices.
Blood culture trivia (61):
1. In adults, each additional milliliter of blood increases recovery by up to 3%.
2. Polymicrobial bacteremias occur 6–18% of the time.
3. Eighty-five percent of coagulase-negative cocci isolated represent contamination. Recent increases in nosocomial septicemia due to these organisms.
4. Fewer anaerobic septicemias in children than in adults.
5. Optimal blood:broth ratio is >1:5.
6. SPS anticoagulant inhibits N. meningitidis, N. gonorrhoeae, G. vaginalis, Streptobacillus spp., Peptostreptococcus, F. tularensis, and M. catarrhalis. Add 1.2% gelatin to counteract the SPS.</td></tr>
<tr><td>Bordetella bronchiseptica
(f. CDC group IVa)
Tiny coccobacillus. Smells awful and grows fast; easily identified by most systems.
This is a mucosal commensal of many animals, e.g., cats, dogs, rabbits, and pigs.</td><td>No CLSI criteria for interpretation. Refer or do MIC only.</td><td><table>
<tr><th></th><th>B. pertussis</th><th>B. parapertussis</th><th>B. bronchiseptica</th></tr>
<tr><td>Regan-Lowe</td><td>+</td><td>+</td><td>+</td></tr>
<tr><td>BA</td><td>–</td><td>+</td><td>+</td></tr>
<tr><td>MacConkey</td><td>–</td><td>–</td><td>+</td></tr>
<tr><td>Oxidase</td><td>+</td><td>–</td><td>+</td></tr>
<tr><td>Catalase</td><td>+</td><td>+</td><td>+</td></tr>
<tr><td>Motile</td><td>–</td><td>–</td><td>+</td></tr>
<tr><td>Urea</td><td>–</td><td>+</td><td>+ (rapid)</td></tr>
</table></td></tr>
<tr><td>Bordetella parapertussis
Nonmotile. Grows better than B. pertussis on Bordet-Gengou medium. Found only in respiratory tract of humans.</td><td>No CLSI criteria for interpretation. Refer or do MIC only.
Rx: aminoglycoside, mezlocillin, piperacillin, ceftazidime, imipenem, and quinolones</td><td>If isolate is inert, motile, and urea positive, think Bordetella.</td></tr>
</table>

Bordetella pertussis	No CLSI criteria for interpretation. Refer or do MIC only. **1st Rx:** erythromycin. Resistance is rare in United States and was first reported in 1994 (30). **2nd Rx:** SXT Close contacts of patients need prophylaxis.	Found only in respiratory tract of humans. No carriers. Minute coccobacillus may need 2-min counterstain. Culture most sensitive in early illness (<2 wk). Confirm with DFA stain: **1.** Use young 24- to 48-h culture. **2.** Excess cells may give false negative DFA stain. Can also do DFA on nasopharynx material. **Serology:** Microagglutination titer may be ordered.
Bordetella hinzii Mostly from chickens and turkeys; also from human respiratory tract, ear, feces. ***Bordetella holmesii*** New species from blood cultures; oxidase negative; nonmotile; brown pigment on heart infusion tyrosine agar. ***Bordetella trematum*** New species from wounds, ear; oxidase negative; motile.	No CLSI criteria for interpretation. Refer or do MIC only.	
Borrelia burgdorferi See Lyme disease (also caused by *B. afzelii* and *B. garinii*)	No CLSI criteria for interpretation. ***B. recurrentis* (relapsing fever)** **1st Rx:** doxycycline **2nd Rx:** erythromycin ***B. burgdorferi* (Lyme disease)** **1st Rx:** ceftriaxone, cefuroxime axetil, doxycycline, amoxicillin **2nd Rx:** penicillin G, cefotaxime Better success if treated early.	Spirochetes detected in skin biopsy specimens collected outside the periphery of the erythema migrans lesion or tissues; stain with Warthin-Starry silver stain or fluorescent antibody stain. Not detected in blood. **Serology:** No antigen tests available. ELISA most commonly used to confirm disease. A titer of 1:256 is positive. May need to confirm with Western blotting. May also order IIF or immunoblotting. Probes are available but are insensitive; PCR is best. Spirochetes grow in Barbour-Stoenner-Kelly II medium in a microaerophilic atmosphere at 30–37°C, incubating for 6 wk.
***Brevibacterium* spp.** Some species may be normal human flora. Ninety percent of human isolates are *B. casei.*	See Diphtheroids. Most MICs for this organism are elevated (36).	Some human isolates give off a distinctive cheeselike odor.
Brevundimonas diminuta ***Brevundimonas vesicularis*** (f. *Pseudomonas diminuta* and *P. vesicularis*)	Do *not* use the disk diffusion test with these organisms. Use a MIC method and interpret with *P. aeruginosa* standards (40).	Unusual in clinical specimens, but *B. diminuta* is associated with few bacteremias. *B. vesicularis* in hemodialysis, sickle cell, and in the immunocompromised. Often requires pantothenate, biotin, and cyanocobalamin vitamins for growth. *B. diminuta* also requires cystine (40).

Organism	Antimicrobic information	Extent of identification and comments
Bronchitis, chronic 10–25% of respiratory tract infections in adults. Bacterial infection implicated in 50–66% of cases. Major agents of chronic disease are *H. influenzae* (nonencapsulated), *M. catarrhalis*, and *S. pneumoniae* (32).	In *chronic* infection, sputum is produced on most days during 3 consecutive mo for more than 2 successive yr. Cigarette smoking, infection, and inhalation of dust or fumes contribute to infection. Most *acute bronchitis* is caused by viral agents such as parainfluenza virus, influenza virus, RSV, adenovirus, or measles virus. Must consider *B. pertussis* in children. Other bacterial causes: *B. pertussis*, *B. parapertussis*, *H. influenzae*, *Mycoplasma pneumoniae*, *Chlamydia pneumoniae*.	
Brucella **spp.**	*Always* refer. Do not test. **1st Rx:** doxycycline + gentamicin or streptomycin **2nd Rx:** doxycycline + rifampin; SXT + gentamicin; chloramphenicol (56)	*Very infectious! Refer out or work in biosafety cabinet only. Alert supervisor.* **Serology:** Slide agglutination test available but should be done in a reference laboratory.
Budvicia aquatica A new member of the *Enterobacteriaceae* mostly from feces and surface water.	K/B, MIC, Etest (interpret with *Enterobacteriaceae* criteria).	Rare in clinical specimens. Lactose negative but becomes positive after 48 h. No etiologic role yet.
Burkholderia cepacia (f. *Pseudomonas cepacia*; CDC EO-1)	MIC or Etest. New K/B standards available for ceftazidime, meropenem, minocycline and SXT (21). **1st Rx:** SXT or meropenem or ciprofloxacin **2nd Rx:** minocycline or chloramphenicol Natural resistance to ampicillin, amoxicillin, narrow-spectrum cephalosporin, colistin, and aminoglycosides (51).	Can smell like *P. aeruginosa*. This is a lysine-positive, oxidase-positive organism (lysine positive is rare in nonfermenters). *S. maltophilia* is lysine positive but oxidase negative. May be yellow on triple sugar iron agar slant. Dangerous nosocomial respiratory pathogen especially in cystic fibrosis, often resistant to quarternary ammonium disinfectants.
Burkholderia gladioli (f. *Pseudomonas gladioli* and *P. marginata*)	Refer or do MIC value only.	Primarily a plant pathogen. Has been reported in sputum from cystic fibrosis patients.
Burkholderia mallei (f. *Pseudomonas mallei*)	Refer. Ensure testing for ceftazidime, tetracycline, and imipenem.	Causes glanders in horses but not in the United States. Can be transmitted to humans. The only nonmotile "pseudomonas" (former name).
Burkholderia pseudomallei (f. *Pseudomonas pseudomallei*)	Refer. Ensure testing for amoxicillin-clavulanic acid, ceftazidime, tetracycline, imipenem, and SXT. **1st Rx:** ceftazidime (intravenous) **2nd Rx:** SXT, imipenem	Melioidosis in humans but not in the United States. Mostly found between 20th parallel north and 20th parallel south. Rough, convoluted colony in 3 days is diagnostic.
Buttiauxella agrestis A new member of the *Enterobacteriaceae* found in water; not a human isolate yet.	Rare, but treat as an enteric with K/B or MIC.	Too rare in humans to worry about. Found in water, soil, snails, slugs. Seven species now. Resembles *Kluyvera*.

Calymmatobacterium granulomatis Causes granuloma inguinale.	Not tested. **1st Rx:** doxycycline **2nd Rx:** erythromycin Lesion must heal before therapy is stopped.	Relapse may occur in 10–20% of patients (66). The disease is characterized by chronic genital ulcers. It is spread by sexual contact. The ulcers may persist for months and may extend into the inguinal region. It is diagnosed by examination of impression smears from biopsy specimens. Wright- or Giemsa-stained smears show clusters of encapsulated bacilli in the cytoplasms of mononuclear cells. These aggregates are called Donovan bodies and are considered diagnostic. The causative organism is morphologically and antigenically similar to *Klebsiella*.
***Campylobacter* spp.** Organisms that may mimic *Campylobacter*: *Aeromonas*, *Pseudomonas* spp., *Vibrio fluvialis*, *Bacillus* spp., *Achromobacter* spp., *Bordetella bronchiseptica*.	No CLSI criteria. Refer if necessary for testing, but resist doing it. Most infections are self-limited and do not require therapy. Susceptibility is predictable. ***C. jejuni*** **1st Rx:** erythromycin **2nd Rx:** fluoroquinolone (some resistance) **3rd Rx:** clindamycin, doxycycline ***C. fetus*** **1st Rx:** imipenem **2nd Rx:** gentamicin **3rd Rx:** ampicillin, chloramphenicol *C. jejuni* and *C. coli* have natural resistance to trimethoprim.	Stool: **1.** Oxidase positive, catalase positive, faint gram-negative rods resembling gull wings. **2.** Growth at 42°C in *Campylobacter* atmosphere. Stinky "Campy"? Think *C. laridis*. Physicians determine therapy based on fever, bloody diarrhea, and >8 stools per day.
Candida albicans **For fungal cultures** Germ tube positive: *Candida albicans* Germ tube negative: yeast identification done **Sterile site, catheter tip, or wound** Germ tube positive: *Candida albicans* Germ tube negative: yeast identification done **Stool: if yeast is 2× the normal flora (44)** Germ tube positive: *Candida albicans* Germ tube negative: *Candida* but not *C. albicans* **Sputum** Rule out *Cryptococcus*; *Candida* is not usually a cause of pneumonia. **Urine** Report: yeast isolated, identification optional.	Resist susceptibility testing. Refer. **Empiric therapy** Bloodstream: amphotericin B or fluconazole Blood, neutropenic: fluconazole Blood, unstable patient: amphotericin B or fluconazole Chronic mucocutaneous: ketoconazole Cutaneous: topical amphotericin B, or clotrimazole, or miconazole, or nystatin Endocarditis: amphotericin B plus flucytosine Thrush, oral (non-AIDS): fluconazole or itraconazole AIDS: stomatitis, esophagitis, vaginitis—fluconazole or itraconazole followed by suppression with fluconazole	Spot test: Gram stain or wet prepn to see budding yeasts. Colonies with "feet" or starlike projections are *C. albicans*! A germ tube interpreted at 3 h is also used if necessary, but never use human serum, and do not incubate >3 h. (20). **Serology:** Serology not reliable although direct antigen tests are available for culture confirmation. Microscopy can be helpful with some yeasts and fungi (7).
Candida*, not *C. albicans Urine or sputum isolates: germ tube negative; blastoconidia produced; pseudohyphae produced. **Yeast, not *C. albicans*** Urine isolates only: germ tube negative; blastoconidia produced; pseudohyphae not produced.	For respiratory isolates, rule out *Cryptococcus* with a urea test. Suspend colony in 3–4 drops of urea broth, incubate 4 h. *Cryptococcus* is positive; *Candida* is negative. Do quality control with each test run.	

Organism	Antimicrobic information	Extent of identification and comments
Capnocytophaga canimorsus (f. DF-2) DF = dysgonic fermenter	No test method available. **1st Rx:** amoxicillin-clavulanate **2nd Rx:** amoxicillin-clavulanate, ciprofloxacin, penicillin G	Needs serum and CO_2; very dangerous in patients, especially those who are splenectomized. Dog bites in splenectomized patients. Does not do well on blood agar initially but observe explosive colony growth after 18 h (key observation).
Capnocytophaga ochracea (f. DF-1)	No test method available. **1st Rx:** clindamycin **2nd Rx:** amoxicillin-clavulanate, ciprofloxacin, penicillin G	See long, thin, wavy gram-negative rods. Oral and periodontal disease, especially in compromised patients. Colony has low, flat, spreading edge and may grow into the agar.
Cardiobacterium hominis	Resist testing or do MIC or try Etest and report only the value. No CLSI criteria available. **1st Rx:** penicillin or ampicillin; gentamicin or tobramycin **2nd Rx:** cefazolin, chloramphenicol, tetracycline	Dangerous in endocarditis. Catalase negative; oxidase positive (unusual reactions for nonfermenters). Normal oral flora. Needs CO_2 and serum for best growth. Pleomorphic and forms rosettes on Gram stain. Susceptible to streptomycin and penicillin.
Cedecea* spp.** Named from where it was discovered: "CDC-e-a." ***Cedecea davisae (f. enteric group 15) ***Cedecea lapagei*** ***Cedecea neteri***	K/B, MIC, or Etest. *Cedecea* spp. are intrinsically resistant to ampicillin, cephalothin, and polymyxin.	Somewhat new *Enterobacteriaceae* isolated from human respiratory specimens and wounds. Lipase positive. *Cedecea* species 3 and 5 not yet named. All species can be tested and reported by CLSI criteria for enterics.
***Cellulomonas* spp.** Name changed to *Cellulosimicrobium*. Usually environmental source.		Most all colonies are pale yellow after 7 days. *Interesting: cellulase activity*—incubate a heavy suspension (McFarland standard of 6) with a piece of sterile copy paper in 0.9% NaCl for 10 days; paper dissolves.
Cellulosimicrobium cellulans (f. *Cellulomonas cellulans* or *Oerskovia xanthineolytica*)		Colonies look a little like *Oerskovia* spp. with its yellowish pigment. The small, thin gram-negative rods are usually motile.
Cerebrospinal fluid isolates	Do *not* report the following antibiotics for any isolate: oral preparations; narrow- and expanded-spectrum cephalosporins except cefuroxime; clindamycin; macrolides; tetracyclines; and fluoroquinolones.	In most cases, CSF collected by lumbar puncture and from shunt meningitis, coagulase-negative staphylococci growing only in broth, not plates, represents skin contamination.

Chlamydia pneumoniae (TWAR) ***Chlamydia psittaci*** TWAR is an outmoded name no longer used for *C. pneumoniae.* TWAR was first designated because two of the original isolates were specified TW-183 and AR-39. Caused a "walking pneumonia" in young adults and college students.	Not tested. **1st Rx:** doxycycline **2nd Rx:** erythromycin; fluoroquinolone Failures occur more often with erythromycin than with doxycycline, but retreatment is often successful (66).	Organisms detected with Giemsa stain and DFA directed against lipopolysaccharide (neither are very good). No molecular tests available. *C. pneumoniae* grows best in HL cells and Hep-2 cells. *C. psittaci* grows best in HeLa, McCoy, and monkey kidney cells. **Serology:** EIA available against lipopolysaccharide should detect all species of *Chlamydia* but is currently licensed only for *C. trachomatis.* Diagnostic test of choice is the species-specific microimmunofluorescence test. Positive diagnosis is IgM of 1:16 and IgG of 1:512 (53).
Chlamydia trachomatis Chlamydia was the most common reportable disease in the United States in 2004, nearly 3 times the frequency reported for gonorrhea.	Not tested. **1st Rx:** doxycycline or azithromycin **2nd Rx:** erythromycin or ofloxacin	Organisms detected with Giemsa and DFA, but DFA is more sensitive; neither stain should be used alone. Molecular tests are available with PCR (best). Can culture in HeLa, McCoy, or monkey kidney cells. **Serology:** Commercial EIA available but less sensitive than culture. Not good in low-prevalence populations. Lymphogranuloma venereum can be diagnosed with a CF titer of >64. Microimmunofluorescence titer should be >32 for IgM or >2,000 for IgG (53).
Chromobacterium violaceum	No test method available. Refer. No CLSI criteria are available for interpretation. **1st Rx:** gentamicin **2nd Rx:** tetracycline, chloramphenicol, SXT Optimal therapy not known.	May or may not have a purple pigment.
Chryseobacterium indologenes (f. *Flavobacterium indologenes*; CDC IIb)	See *Flavobacterium indologenes.*	
Chryseobacterium meningosepticum (f. *Flavobacterium meningosepticum*; CDC IIa)	See *Flavobacterium meningosepticum.* **1st Rx:** vancomycin +/– rifampin **2nd Rx:** ciprofloxacin, levofloxacin	
Chryseomonas luteola (f. Ve-1; *Pseudomonas luteola*)	No test method available. Try MIC or Etest value only.	Yellow pigmented and oxidase negative is a hint. Also see wrinkled colony. Very similar to *Flavimonas oryzihabitans* (Ve-2), which is arginine negative 86% of the time.
Citrobacter amalonaticus (f. *Levinea amalonatica*) ***Citrobacter koseri*** (f. *Citrobacter diversus*) ***C. braakii*** ***C. farmeri*** ***C. sedlakii*** ***Citrobacter* species 10** ***Citrobacter* species 11** ***C. werkmanii*** ***C. youngae*** ***Citrobacter freundii***	K/B, MIC, Etest. All CLSI interpretive criteria are valid for enterics. May develop resistance during prolonged therapy with third-generation cephalosporins; therefore, retest susceptible isolates within 3–4 days after initiation of therapy (21). ***C. diversus* and *C. freundii*** **1st Rx:** imipenem or meropenem **2nd Rx:** fluoroquinolone	First, distinguish colonization from infection. Always report AMP as resistant for *C. amalonaticus*, i.e., it is intrinsically resistant. *C. freundii* is always resistant to cephalothin. *C. diversus* is always resistant to cephalothin and carbenicillin (27).

Organism	Antimicrobic information	Extent of identification and comments
Cladosporium More than 30 species. The most common are *C. elatum*, *C. herbarum*, *C. sphaerospermum*, *and C. cladosporioides.*	No data on susceptibility profiles. **Rx:** itraconazole	A dematiaceous mold usually considered a contaminant but that has been isolated from skin and nail infection, keratitis, and sinusitis. Use a biosafety level 2 safety cabinet for manipulation. Tissue may contain brown hyphae.
Clonorchis See Trematodes		
Clostridium difficile Test for toxin A and B.		Process up to three specimens, one per 24-h period. Once a test is positive, stop testing. Further positives have no meaning. The negative predictive value of the first stool specimen is 97%. Do not do a *C. difficile* toxin test for a test of cure. Testing formed stools is usually unproductive unless there are >30,000 white blood cells present in hospitalized patients.
CMV See Cytomegalovirus		
Coccidioides	**1st Rx:** fluconazole or amphotericin B **2nd Rx:** itraconazole	May appear as a tan, matte colony rather than white and fluffy. Arthroconidia are highly infectious but may not appear in culture until after 4–5 days of growth. Grows well on *Legionella* media. **Serology:** Immunity develops after infection. Skin test positive about a month after onset. May request complement fixation, double diffusion, or latex agglutination to detect antibodies.
Comamonas acidovorans (f. *Pseudomonas acidovorans*) ***Comamonas terrigena*** Rare in humans. ***Comamonas testosteroni*** (f. *Pseudomonas testosteroni*)	No test method available. Try MIC or Etest value only.	Motile by flagellar tufts on polar stalks. Primarily a soil (environment) organism. *C. testosteroni* is inert, oxidase-positive, catalase-positive, gram-negative rods recovered from sputum, peritoneal fluid, urine, and stool. Uncertain pathogenicity of either. Orange indole reaction due to anthranilic acid from tryptone.
Conidiobolus Several species, the most common of which are *C. coronatus*, *C. incongruus*, and *C. lamprauges.*	Submit to reference laboratory for testing. In vivo response to therapy not well documented.	A fungus occasionally involved in nasal and facial infection; causes a chronic, inflammatory granulomatous disease called entomophthoromycosis conidiobolae.
Conjunctivitis The most common of the eye infections.	Site of infection in the eye correlates to certain pathogens. In children, common causes are *H. influenzae*, *S. pneumoniae*, and *S. aureus.* Twenty percent of cases in children and 14% in adults are due to adenovirus types 4, 3, and 7A and are highly contagious.	

Corynebacterium spp. (diphtheroids) (36) **Associated infections:** ***C. aquaticum*** See *Leifsonia* (meningitis, peritonitis) ***C. diphtheriae*** Pharynx, nasal, skin ***C. minutissimum*** Erythrasma, bacteremia ***C. pseudotuberculosis*** Lymphadenitis, pneumonia ***C. jeikeium*** (JK) See below (septicemia, meningitis, peritonitis, catheter or foreign body infections) ***C. urealyticum*** See below (cystitis, systemic, skin, catheter associated) ***C. striatum*** Normal skin flora ***C. ulcerans*** Pharyngitis; may produce toxin, like *C. diphtheriae.* Note: organisms that grow better on blood than chocolate are *C. jeikeium*, *Corynebacterium* group G-2, *Arcanobacterium*, and *S. pneumoniae.*	The Etest may be used for AST to report MIC value only. *C. diphtheriae*: antitoxin given to patients with laryngeal or pharyngeal disease. **1st Rx:** erythromycin **2nd Rx:** clindamycin	Classic genus characteristics (22, 62): **1.** Pleomorphic, club-shaped, gram-positive rods ("Chinese letters" on some media) **2.** No true branching **3.** Catalase positive **4.** Nonmotile **5.** Aerobic growth better than anaerobic growth **6.** Opaque white or gray colony **7.** Esculin negative If recovered from nonsterile site, do Gram stain and catalase. Consider to be a commensal if other commensals present. Identification optional: do only if white blood cells are present and physician requests. **Serology:** Not used in diagnosis of diphtheria, but can be used to measure immunity by neutralization tests. If recovered from sterile site, identify by request using special corynebacterium identification system. Even CDC has difficulty identifying all diphtheroids to species level. If from ear, consider *Turicella otitidis* (see chart). *Corynebacterium ulcerans* causes a zoonotic infection similar to diphtheria but no person-to-person transmission. Studies indicate that signs and symptoms of a diphtheria-like illness caused by *C. ulcerans* are milder than those caused by *C. diphtheriae*. However, some strains of *C. ulcerans* produce potent diphtheria toxin and may cause severe symptoms similar to those caused by *C. diphtheriae.*
Corynebacterium jeikeium (f. *Corynebacterium* JK)	**1st Rx:** vancomycin **2nd Rx:** penicillin G + antipseudomonal aminoglycoside May require removal of catheter for cure. Always confirm if resistant to vancomycin, teicoplanin, or linezolid.	Often associated with septicemia and indwelling catheters. Also skin; endocarditis and pneumonia; may be multiply resistant. Slow-growing, catalase-positive diphtheroid often susceptible only to vancomycin. Identify with commercial system with this organism in its database.

Organism	Antimicrobic information	Extent of identification and comments
Corynebacterium urealyticum (group D2)	Resist testing if possible. Etest for value only. **1st Rx:** vancomycin or teicoplanin **2nd Rx:** doxycycline	Urine: **1.** Slow growing, opaque, smooth, convex, nonhemolytic. May need 72 h for colony development. **2.** Catalase positive, diphtheroid; may be short rods. **3.** Urea slant positive in <15 min. **4.** Urine usually shows elevated pH (~8) with packed red blood cells and struvite crystals (ammonium magnesium phosphate) suggestive of encrusted cystitis (36). Infections: cystitis; systemic; skin; catheters. Risk factors: hospitalized, urologically manipulated, elderly. Significant underlying disease: immunosupression; urology surgery; prior antibiotic therapy (65).
Corynebacterium xerosis	Same as *C. urealyticum* above.	
Coxiella burnetii ☣	No CLSI criteria. Unable to test. **1st Rx:** doxycycline (acute disease); ciprofloxacin or doxycycline + rifampin (chronic disease) **2nd Rx:** erythromycin (acute disease); fluoroquinolone + doxycycline for 3 yr (chronic disease)	Causes Q fever. Can inhale aerosols or ingest unpasteurized dairy products. Organism can be cultured in monkey kidney, Vero, and human embryonic fibroblast cell lines and in egg yolk sacs or in animals, but culture is rarely done. Serology is the diagnostic test of choice; IFA is recommended. Consider a fourfold rise in titer or a phase II antibody titer of ≥256 to be diagnostic. Phase I antibody titers are usually higher than phase II titers in chronic infection. DFA is available but has poor sensitivity (12).
Critical values See Panic values		
Cryptococcus neoformans ☣	Do not test.	Urease positive, often within 30 min of inoculating. Use this to quickly rule out *Cryptococcus* from other yeasts from respiratory specimens. Spot test: spherical, budding yeast. Nonpigmented colonies on Sabouraud agar or BA and may or may not be mucoid. A rapid (30 min–4 h) phenol oxidase test by commercial disk identifies this isolate at 95% accuracy (20). **Serology:** Latex agglutination detects antigen. Tests for antibodies not often used to monitor patients.
Cryptosporidium parvum Recognized in 1976. Acute, self-limiting diarrhea, lasting 7–14 days and accompanied by nausea, cramps, and low fever. More severe in AIDS patients.	Do not test. No effective treatment to date.	Incidence of ~2% in AIDS patients. *Cryptosporidium* is diagnosed in 10–20% of AIDS patients with diarrhea in hospital-based studies. *Cryptosporidium* is not killed by chlorine in drinking water. Must boil water for 1 full minute.
CSF isolates See Cerebrospinal fluid isolates		
Curtobacterium Six species are recognized. Very rare in humans. Usually plant (e.g., rice) pathogens.	Refer for testing if required.	Small, short coryneform rods with no branching. Catalase positive and usually motile. May be creamy, yellow, or orange pigmented.

Curvularia *C. lunata* is the most prevalent species in humans and animals, but there are several other species in the genus.	No standardized procedure available for susceptibility testing. Refer to reference lab. Amphotericin B, itraconazole, and terbinafine have been used, but the prognosis is usually poor, particularly for immunocompromised patients.	A dematiaceous, filamentous, olive-brown-to-black fungus normally found in nature and as a laboratory contaminant but that may cause human illness, mostly in eyes and sinus. Mycetoma and phaeohyphomycosis at various sites including brain and lungs.
Cyclospora cayetanensis	**1st Rx:** SXT	Outbreaks of this parasite have been traced to fruits (various "berries") contaminated with human sewage, and it has been suggested that many cases of "traveler's diarrhea" might be caused by this parasite. It is diagnosed by finding oocysts in the patient's fecal material. Symptoms associated with this parasite are variable and vague.
Cytomegalovirus (CMV) A member of the herpesvirus family.	For now, there are no treatments for pregnant women whose fetuses might be infected with CMV. Current drugs that are effective against CMV have serious side effects and are not approved for use in pregnant women. There is some evidence that ganciclovir may prevent hearing loss in infants born with congenital CMV. However, this drug has serious side effects and was tested only in children with severe congenital CMV symptoms. Resistance testing by gene sequencing of the UL97 or UL54 gene can be ordered from some reference labs.	CDC data indicate that between 50% and 80% of adults in the United States are infected with CMV by 40 years of age. CMV is the most common virus transmitted to a pregnant woman's unborn child. Approximately 1 in 150 children is born with congenital CMV infection. Approximately 1 in 750 children is born with or develops permanent disabilities due to CMV. The virus is found in body fluids, including urine, saliva (spit), breast milk, blood, tears, semen, and vaginal fluids. Once CMV is in a person's body, it stays there for life. Most CMV infections are "silent," meaning they cause no signs or symptoms in an infected person. Transmission of CMV occurs from person to person, through close contact with body fluids (urine, saliva, breast milk, blood, tears, semen, and vaginal fluids), but the chance of getting CMV infection from casual contact is very small. **Serology:** Diagnose by IIF (IgM and IgG), ELISA (IgM and IgG), passive hemagglutination (PHA) available in reference labs.
Delftia **spp.**	No CLSI criteria available for testing.	Phenotypically like *Comamonas*, but oxidize fructose and mannitol. Twenty-five percent have fluorescent pigment and 50% may be yellow or tan. Isolates are oxidase positive and grow on MacConkey agar.
Dengue virus	No specific therapy.	A flavivirus transmitted by mosquitoes. WHO estimates about 50,000,000 infections worldwide, which is about 95 cases per minute.
Dermabacter **spp.** Usually reported as diphtheroid. Normal human skin flora.	See Diphtheroids. *D. hominis* may be resistant to aminoglycosides (36).	Often mistaken for small-colony coagulase-negative staphylococci. Are coccobacillary or coccoid on Gram stain, which is unusual and characteristic. May need special corynebacterium systems to identify.
Dermatophytes	One of three genera (*Microsporum*, *Trichophyton*, and *Epidermophyton*) causing hair, skin, and nail infections.	
Diphtheroids Usually reported based on colony morphology and Gram stain. Referred to as coryneforms also.	No CLSI guidelines for coryneforms. Do MIC with Etest or microdilution, reporting a value only. Can do disk diffusion with Mueller-Hinton + 5% sheep's blood using streptococcus interpretive criteria (report which interpretations you use). May include *Arcanobacterium*, *Arthrobacter*, *Brevibacterium*, *Cellulomonas*, *Cellulosimicrobium*, *Corynebacterium*, *Curtobacterium*, *Dermabacter*, *Exiguobacterium*, *Leifsonia*, *Microbacterium*, *Oerskovia*, *Rothia*, and/or *Turicella* (22, 36).	

Organism	Antimicrobic information	Extent of identification and comments
Dolosicocccus paucivorans (63)		Gram-positive coccus. Only isolates have been from a blood culture from elderly patient with pneumonia. Uncertain significance. PYR positive, LAP negative, vancomycin susceptible, NaCl negative.
Dysgonomonas Includes *D. capnocytophagoides* (f. DF-3) and *D. gadei.* Closer to *Bacteroides forsythus* and *B. distasonis* than to *Capnocytophaga.*	Refer for testing. Usually resistant to beta-lactams, aminoglycosides, macrolides, and quinolones. Susceptible to tetracycline, imipenem, rifampin, and SXT (75).	Coccoid, small gram-negative rods whose colonies smell like strawberries (75). Require enriched media, facultative slow growth, nonmotile. *D. capnocytophagoides*: mostly from stools of immunocompromised patients. *D. gadei*: one isolate from gallbladder.
Ear infections (31)	**Causes of otitis externa** Acute: *S. aureus*, *S. pyogenes*; *P. aeruginosa*; gram-negative rods Chronic: *P. aeruginosa*; anaerobes **Causes of otitis media** Acute: *S. pneumoniae* (33%); *H. influenzae* (20%); *S. pyogenes* (8%); RSV; influenza virus (viral = 4%) Chronic: anaerobes	
EBV See Epstein-Barr virus		
Echoviruses Name derived from their initial description: enteric cytopathogenic human orphan.		Includes coxsackieviruses, echoviruses, hepatitis A virus, and poliovirus. Enterovirus 70 is associated with conjunctivitis and enterovirus 71 is associated with encephalitis in humans.
Edwardsiella tarda	K/B, MIC, Etest with enteric criteria. Therapy for gastroenteritis may not be indicated.	Mostly from cold-blooded animals. Opportunistic in humans.
EF-4a and EF-4b EF-4a is similar to *Pasteurella*, often from dogs. EF-4b is often from cats.	Refer for testing. EF-4a: variable to penicillin and resistant to clindamycin and trimethoprim.	Both are normal oral flora of dogs, cats, and rodents. EF-4a: some yellow pigment, coccoid gram-negative rods, mousy-popcorn smell, nonmotile, arginine positive, causing usually local infections. EF-4b: coccoid, popcorn smell, nonpigmented, arginine negative.
Ehrlichia spp. *Ehrlichia chaffeensis* *Ehrlichia phagocytophila*	Tests not done. **1st Rx:** doxycycline **2nd Rx:** tetracycline or rifampin	Peripheral blood (best) or spinal fluid inoculated into specific cell lines can be used for culture, but it is rarely done. Takes >1 mo. IFA is the most commonly used test. See a fourfold titer rise in paired sera or a peak titer of ≥64 (for *E. chaffeensis*). *Amblyomma americanum* (Lone Star tick) or *Dermacentor variabilis* (American dog tick) spreads both *E. chaffeensis* and *E. ewingii.*
Eikenella corrodens (f. HB-1)	No test method available. Do not test. Resistant to clindamycin, cephalexin, erythromycin, and metronidazole. **1st Rx:** penicillin G, ampicillin, or amoxicillin-clavulanate **2nd Rx:** SXT, fluoroquinolone Add aminoglycoside for endocarditis cases (66).	Fastidious, needs CO_2. Catalase negative, oxidase positive is unusual for nonfermenters. Smells like mushrooms or like chlorine bleach. Normal in upper respiratory tract. Found in human scratches and bites, blood, CSF.

Empedobacter brevis (f. *Flavobacterium breve*) See *Flavobacterium breve*	No CLSI criteria. Refer or MIC value or Etest value only.	
Endocarditis, infective Infection of the endocardium commonly caused by bacteria. Endothelial surface damage from catheters or congenital problems provides a site for bacterial adhesion. Coagulase-negative staphylococcus true infection is fairly common in patients on central venous catheters. *S. epidermidis* most common on prosthetic valves. *S. aureus* is second most common. Common in native valve: viridans group streptococci, enterococci, *S. aureus*. Less common: *Abiotrophia*, *Streptococcus bovis*, coagulase-negative staphylococci, enterics, *Pseudomonas* (especially in drug abusers), *Haemophilus*, unusual gram-negative bacteria, yeast (5, 8, 45).		
Enterobacter aerogenes ***Enterobacter agglomerans*** (current name is *Pantoea agglomerans*) ***Enterobacter asburiae*** (f. enteric group 17) ***Enterobacter cloacae*** ***Enterobacter gergoviae*** ***Enterobacter hormaechei*** (f. enteric group 75) ***Enterobacter sakazakii*** Causes meningitis in children; yellow pigmented ***Enterobacter cancerogenus* (*taylorae*)** (f. enteric group 19)	CLSI criteria used as per *Enterobacteriaceae*. K/B, MIC, Etest using enteric criteria. **1st Rx:** ertapenem, imipenem, or meropenem or antipseudomonals; penicillin + antipseudomonals; aminoglycoside **2nd Rx:** ticarcillin-clavulanate or piperacillin-tazobactam or ciprofloxacin *E. cloacae* and *E. aerogenes* are intrinsically resistant to cephalothin.	Generally one should *not* see susceptibility to ampicillin, cefazolin, or cephalothin with *Enterobacter* spp. May develop resistance during prolonged therapy with broad spectrum cephalosporins; therefore retest susceptible isolates within 3–4 days after initiation of therapy (21).
***Enterobius vermicularis* (pinworm)**	**1st Rx:** pyrantel pamoate or mebendazole **2nd Rx:** albendazole	Pinworms are very contagious! The female crawls out of the anus (causing itching) and lays her eggs directly on the perianal skin. Bed linens, clothing, carpets, etc., can be contaminated with eggs. The infected person's hands will be contaminated with eggs, providing a route for reinfection and egg dispersal. Therefore, if one member of a family is infected, the whole family must be treated. Pinworm and *Dientamoeba* infections may occur simultaneously, since *Dientamoeba* may be found within pinworm eggs.
***Enterococcus* spp.** Most common: *E. faecalis*. Likely resistant to ampicillin: *E. faecium*.	Always confirm if resistant to both ampicillin and quinupristin-dalfopristin, or to teicoplanin but not vancomycin. If *E. faecium* is resistant to ampicillin, it is probably *E. faecalis*, so confirm the identification. *Antimicrobials that should never be reported:* cephalosporins; clindamycin; SXT; aminoglycosides (except high concentrations) because in vitro results do not correlate to in vivo response (21).	Enterococci are PYR positive, LAP positive, bile esculin positive, and NaCl positive. Confirm Gram stain and catalase negative. *Enterococcus*, group A streptococcus, nutritionally variant streptococcus (*Abiotrophia*), and *Aerococcus* spp. are 95–100% PYR positive.

Organism	Antimicrobic information	Extent of identification and comments
Enterovirus This group includes the polioviruses, coxsackieviruses, echoviruses, and other enteroviruses. In addition to the three different polioviruses, there are 62 nonpolio enteroviruses that can cause disease in humans: 23 coxsackie A viruses, 6 coxsackie B viruses, 28 echoviruses, and 5 other enteroviruses.	No vaccine is currently available for the nonpolio enteroviruses, and no specific therapy exists.	Enteroviruses are small RNA viruses. Nonpolio enteroviruses are very common. CDC data suggest that they are second only to the "common cold" viruses (the rhinoviruses) as the most common viral infectious agents in humans. The enteroviruses cause an estimated 10–15 million or more symptomatic infections a year in the United States. All three types of polioviruses have been eliminated from the western hemisphere, as well as the western Pacific and European regions, by the widespread use of vaccines. Most infections are asymptomatic. Those who do become ill usually develop either mild upper respiratory symptoms (a "summer cold"), a flulike illness with fever and muscle aches, or an illness with rash.
Epidermophyton Causes ringworm. *E. floccosum* is the only species (of two) that is pathogenic in humans.	No standard methods available. Terbinafine, itraconazole, and ketoconazole have been used successfully.	One of the dermatophytes that produces infection of the skin and nails, but not hair. Causes athlete's foot, jock itch, and ringworm of the body. Produces only macroconidia; the other dermatophytes produce microconidia and macroconidia.
Epstein-Barr virus A member of the herpesvirus family that causes infectious mononucleosis and is associated with nasopharyngeal carcinoma and Burkitt's lymphoma.		**Serology:** Infection leads to formation of heterophile antibodies in persons >4 yr old. Transmitted by infected saliva, hence the "kissing disease" term. Heterophile monospot test detects primary, early, and some past infections. IgM to viral capsid antigen detects primary and early infection. IgG to viral capsid antigen detects primary, early, past, and reactivation infections. Early antigen and Epstein-Barr nuclear antigen may also be useful.
Erwinia amylovora New member of the *Enterobacteriaceae* associated with plant diseases.	Test not necessary.	Not associated with human specimens. If isolated, it will likely be environmentally associated. Pathogenicity for humans unlikely unless from a sterile site.
Erysipelothrix rhusiopathiae Gram-positive rod that can easily destain and appear gram negative. H_2S in triple sugar iron agar looks like an upside-down feather along the stab line.	**1st Rx:** penicillin or ampicillin **2nd Rx:** fluoroquinolone or broad-spectrum cephalosporin Intrinsic resistance to vancomycin and aminoglycosides.	Not part of normal human flora. Is an animal organism and is seen in people who have or work with animals. Causes erysipeloid, a painful, local skin infection. Can identify with some *Corynebacterium* identification kits. Catalase-negative, gram-positive rod.
ESBL See Extended-spectrum beta-lactamase (21)		

Escherichia coli (common)	K/B, MIC, Etest. **1st Rx:** beta-lactams and beta-lactam inhibitor combinations, a fluoroquinolone, SXT, imipenem, depending on site	Strains that produce ESBLs may be clinically resistant to therapy with penicillins, cephalosporin, or aztreonam despite apparent in vitro susceptibility to some of these agents. See Extended-spectrum beta-lactamase below for test criteria and interpretations. *Escherichia* is genetically the same as *Shigella.* Use spot test where possible: lactose positive on MacConkey plate, spot indole positive from BA and beta-hemolytic will provide 95% confidence. No need to reconfirm with another method. If the isolate is lactose positive and nonhemolytic and PYR negative, it is also *E. coli* (20).
***Escherichia coli* A-D (Alkalescens-Dispar group)**	K/B, MIC, Etest. Therapy same as for common *E. coli.*	Looks like a shigella, but serology negative.
***Escherichia coli* O157:H7** Use sorbitol-MacConkey plate (*this organism is sorbitol negative and colorless on the agar*). Other sorbitol-negative common enterics: Some *Cedecea* spp. *Edwardsiella* Some *Enterobacter* spp. Some *Shigella* spp. *Proteus* *Providencia* *Pragia* Therefore, confirm with serology.	AST should not be reported without direct consult with clinician. *Therapy for O157 infection has not been demonstrated to be efficacious and safe, except for cases of cystitis and pyelonephritis.* Therefore, AST is only useful for epidemiologic purposes (10, 21). 95% resolve; 5% develop hemolytic-uremic syndrome. Shiga toxin is on the select agent list.	If identified as sorbitol negative by plate or by instrument, set up O157 latex test. Report: If a positive test occurs, report as "*E. coli* serogroup O157, referred to reference lab for O157:H7 confirmation." Disease characteristics: Diarrhea, 93% Abdominal cramps, 79% Bloody stool, 39–63% Slight or no fever, 16–45% Highest yield: <6 days of onset (15) Some laboratories test for Shiga-like toxin from broth and submit positive broth to a reference laboratory for culture.
Escherichia fergusonii (f. enteric group 10)	K/B, MIC, Etest. Use CLSI criteria for enterics.	Opportunistic: from blood and spinal fluid.
Escherichia hermanii	K/B, MIC, Etest. Use CLSI criteria for enterics. Intrinsically resistant to ampicillin and carbapenem (27).	
Escherichia vulneris	K/B, MIC, Etest. Use CLSI criteria for enterics.	Human wounds.
Ewingella americana (f. enteric group 40) New member of the *Enterobacteriaceae* isolated from respiratory tract and blood. No environmental source known.	K/B, MIC, Etest. Use CLSI criteria for enterics. Intrinsically resistant to cephalothin (27).	Similar to *Cedecea* but lipase negative.
Exophiala *E. jeanselmei* currently has two varieties: *E. jeanselmei* var. *heteromorpha* and *E. jeanselmei* var. *lecanii-corni.* Other common isolates are *E. castellanii, E. moniliae, E. pisciphila, E. salmonis,* and *E. spinifera.*	Submit to reference laboratory for testing. Amphotericin B with or without flucytosine, itraconazole, and terbinafine have been used.	A dematiaceous fungus saprophytic in nature but that causes infections in humans as phaeohyphomycosis. Appears in tissue as brown hyphae and yeastlike cells. *E. dermatitidis* and *Wangiella dermatitidis* are taxonomically close and may be interchanged by some.

Organism	Antimicrobic information	Extent of identification and comments
Exserohilum The common clinical species include *E. rostratum* and *E. longirostratum.*	Refer for susceptibility testing. Few data available.	A dematiaceous, filamentous fungus common in grass and soil. May rarely cause human cutaneous and subcutaneous infection.
Extended-spectrum beta-lactamase (ESBL) (21) (for *K. pneumoniae*, *K. oxytoca*, *Proteus mirabilis*, and *E. coli*) *P. mirabilis* should be screened only when from blood culture. ESBL-positive strains may be clinically resistant to therapy with all penicillins, cephalosporins, or aztreonam regardless of in vitro results and should be reported as resistant.	*MIC test procedure: Screen* using standard MIC procedure. A positive ESBL screen for ceftazidime (1 μg/ml), aztreonam (1), cefotaxime (1), and ceftriaxone (1) would exhibit a MIC of ≥2. Cefpodoxime (4 μg/ml) would have a MIC of ≥8. *Confirm* using: ceftazidime (0.25–128) + ceftazidime-clavulanate (0.25/4–128/4) and cefotaxime (0.25–64) + cefotaxime-clavulanate (0.25/4–64/4 μg/ml). A ≥3 twofold decrease in MIC for either agent in combination with clavulanate confirms ESBL. Control with *E. coli* ATCC 25922 and *K. pneumoniae* ATCC 700603.	
***Facklamia* spp.** Closely related to *Globicatella*. There are four species in the genus.		A gram-positive coccus. Isolated from blood, wounds, and urinary sites (63). Catalase negative, PYR positive, LAP positive, NaCl positive, esculin negative, vancomycin susceptible.
Fasciola See Trematodes		
Fasciolopsis See Trematodes		
Fifth disease Caused by parvovirus B19. Also called erythema infectiosum. The human virus is different from the animal parvovirus and humans cannot be infected with the animal virus. Historically, the six common rash illnesses were "counted" as measles (first disease), scarlet fever (second), rubella (third, German measles), a rash illness still called Duke's disease or fourth disease, fifth disease, and roseola (sixth disease).	No vaccine is available for this disease.	CDC describes fifth disease as a mild, contagious rash illness that occurs most commonly in children 5–15 yr old. The ill child typically has a "slapped-cheek" rash on the face and a lacy red rash on the trunk and limbs that may itch. An ill child may have a low-grade fever, malaise, or a "cold" a few days before the rash breaks out. The child is usually not very ill, and the rash resolves in 7 to 10 days. Parvovirus B19 may cause a serious illness in persons with sickle-cell disease or similar types of chronic anemia.
Flavimonas oryzihabitans See *Pseudomonas oryzihabitans.*		
Flavobacterium breve Now called *Empedobacter brevis.*	MIC value or Etest value only. Disk test unreliable. Most flavobacteria are naturally resistant to ampicillin, amoxicillin, and narrow-spectrum cephalosporins.	Catalase positive, oxidase positive, indole positive; slight yellow pigment. Nonmotile; grows best at 30°C.

Flavobacterium gleum (f. IIb) Strong yellow pigment.		Catalase positive, oxidase positive, indole positive (extraction). Cells may look like dumbbells, thus the "II" designation.
Flavobacterium indologenes (f. IIb) Now called *Chryseobacterium indologenes.*		
Flavobacterium meningosepticum (f. IIa) Now called *Chryseobacterium meningosepticum.* Slight yellow pigment.		In newborns and premature infants and in nurseries. Environmental. Catalase positive, oxidase positive, indole positive (extraction). Cells pulled in the middle to look like dumbbells.
Flavobacterium multivorum (f. IIK-2) Now called *Sphingobacterium multivorum.*		An indole-negative *Flavobacterium*. Slight yellow pigment. Similar biochemically to *Pseudomonas paucimobilis* except *Flavobacterium* is nonmotile.
Flavobacterium odoratum (f. M-4f) Now called *Myroides odoratus.*		An indole-negative flavobacterium. Fruity odor (apples). Spreading edge to colony. Most CDC isolates have been from urine. Inert biochemistry.
Flavobacterium spiritivorum See *Sphingobacterium spiritivorum*		An indole-negative *Flavobacterium*. Slight yellow pigment.
Other *Flavobacterium* spp.		
Fonsecaea The two recognized species are *F. compacta* and *F. pedrosoi.*	Submit to reference laboratory for testing. Itraconazole may be used in conjunction to surgical removal. Therapy may or may not be successful.	A dematiaceous, filamentous fungus (in culture) that causes chromoblastomycosis with lesions usually in subcutaneous tissue of legs or feet but can occur in the nose. One commonly sees in tissues sclerotic bodies that are dark brown, spherical or polyhedral, thick-walled structures which have horizontal and vertical septa inside.
Francisella tularensis *Highly virulent and infectious! If suspicious, put into safety cabinet and prepare to send out.*	Refer for testing. **1st Rx:** streptomycin or gentamicin or tobramycin **2nd Rx:** doxycycline or ciprofloxacin (for postexposure prophylaxis) Relapse may occur unless an aminoglycoside is used.	Stop handling and refer for identification if very tiny gram-negative coccobacillus from blood, lymph node aspirate, or respiratory specimens. Blood isolates that will grow slowly on chocolate agar but poorly or not at all on blood agar in 24 h. Faint growth in thioglycolate; requires cysteine in other broth. Confirmed with DFA.
Fusarium More than 20 species, the most common of which are *F. solani* (the most virulent), *F. oxysporum*, and *F. chlamydosporum.*	Submit to reference laboratory for testing. *Fusarium* infections are difficult to treat, and the invasive forms can be fatal. Amphotericin B alone or in combination with flucytosine or rifampin is the most commonly used antifungal drug for treatment of systemic disease. Voriconazole may be used also.	A filamentous fungus that is a common contaminant and plant pathogen but an emerging opportunistic pathogen in humans. Both cutaneous and systemic infections have occurred. Mycotoxins may be produced and contaminate grains. Macroconidia are multicelled, canoe-shaped and pointed.

Organism	Antimicrobic information	Extent of identification and comments
Gardnerella vaginalis SPS is inhibitory.	Do not test. **1st Rx:** metronidazole **2nd Rx:** clindamycin	Gram variable, catalase negative, growth on chocolate agar better than on BA. This organism is not necessarily an indicator of vaginitis or vaginosis. These conditions are best diagnosed by microscopy, not culture. Male sex partner need not be treated.
Gemella* spp.** ***G. morbillorum (f. *Streptococcus morbillorum*) Cells in pairs or chains. ***G. haemolysans*** Cells in pairs or clusters (may look like a neisseria with flat sides). ***G. bergeri* and *G. sanguinis*** Less common and significance less understood. Cells in pairs or chains.	MIC value or Etest value only. Usually susceptible to penicillin, chloramphenicol, vancomycin, streptomycin, erythromycin (13% R), and tetracycline (7% R).	Gram-positive cocci. Alpha- or nonhemolytic. Easily decolorized in Gram stain. Catalase negative, vancomycin susceptible, PYR positive, LAP positive, bile esculin negative, NaCl negative (*Leuconostoc* and *Pediococcus* are vancomycin resistant).
Geotrichum The most common species is *G. candidum*. *Geotrichum clavatum* and *Geotrichum fici* (which smells like pineapple) may also be reported.	Disseminated geotrichosis has a poor prognosis and a 75% mortality rate. Therapy with amphotericin B with or without flucytosine has been used as has itraconazole.	A yeastlike organism that causes geotrichosis of lungs, mouth, intestines, and vagina of compromised patients but can also be normal human intestinal flora. Hyphae segment into arthroconidia. Colonies may resemble ground glass.
Giardia lamblia Several *Giardia* species exist, but *G. lamblia* is the most common in humans in the United States. Some refer to it as *G. intestinalis*.	**1st Rx:** tinidazole **2nd Rx:** metronidazole	*G. lamblia* trophozoites live in the small intestine of the host. Cysts are passed in the feces of an infected host and the next host is infected when it ingests cysts in contaminated food or water. Rather than being invasive, the trophozoites adhere to the lining of the small intestine and millions can be passed daily. Wilderness streams may also be a source of the organism.
***Globicatella* spp.**	MIC value or Etest value only.	Gram-positive cocci in chains; vancomycin susceptible, PYR positive, LAP negative, bile esculin negative, NaCl positive.
***Gordonia* spp.** (f. *Gordona* or *Rhodococcus*) Aerobic actinomycetes. Thirteen total species, but only five species isolated from humans.	No CLSI criteria. Refer. **1st Rx:** erythromycin or rifampin, ciprofloxacin, gentamicin, vancomycin, or imipenem	Diphtheroid-like or coccobacillus. Colony growth appears as coccobacilli in zigzag configuration (similar to *Tsukamurella*). Nonhemolytic, mucoid colonies that may become salmon pink. Susceptible to lysozyme, urea positive, and nitrate positive.
***Granulicatella* spp.** Like *Abiotrophia*, previously known as nutritionally variant or satelliting streptococcus and includes the former *A. adiacens* and *A. elegans* as the two species in the genus (63).	No CLSI criteria.	

HACEK *Haemophilus aphrophilus*, *Actinobacillus* spp., *Cardiobacterium hominis*, *Eikenella corrodens*, *Kingella* spp.	Commercial identification systems not reliable. No CLSI criteria for interpretation of MIC (do not use disk test for these slow growers). Report Etest or MIC value without interpretations.	These are relatively fastidious organisms capable of causing endocarditis and when isolated from blood culture should be quickly reported.
Haemophilus aphrophilus	See *H. influenzae.* No CLSI criteria. Typically resistant to vancomycin, clindamycin, and methicillin. **1st Rx:** (penicillin or ampicillin) or (ampicillin-sulbactam) +/– gentamicin **2nd Rx:** expanded- or broad-spectrum cephalosporin + gentamicin	Small coccoid cells similar to *Capnocytophaga*. Needs CO_2 but not X or V factors. May appear granular in broth, first on side of bottle or on surface. May take 5–7 days for growth. Acid/acid in triple sugar iron agar slant. Do cefinase for beta-lactamase.
Haemophilus ducreyi	See *H. influenzae.* **1st Rx:** azithromycin or ceftriaxone **2nd Rx:** erythromycin or ciprofloxacin Sexual contacts should be treated.	Requires X, not V. Colonies can be pushed around on plate. See cells in parallel chains or swirls. Causes soft chancre, a painful sexually transmitted disease. Requires chocolate agar (GC base) + 3 µg/ml vancomycin to isolate from lesions.
Haemophilus haemolyticus	See *H. influenzae.* Do cefinase only.	Probably not pathogenic. Rare in nasopharynx. X and V required.
Haemophilus influenzae Requires X and V. At least six biotypes.	Use CLSI *Haemophilus* criteria for K/B or MIC with *Haemophilus* test medium. For blood and CSF isolates, report only AMP, a broad-spectrum cephalosporin, chloramphenicol, and meropenem (21). Disk test and MIC test require special media for testing. **Sterile site and serious illness** **1st Rx:** cefotaxime, ceftriaxone **2nd Rx:** SXT, imipenem, fluoroquinolones **Other sites, (throat, respiratory, etc.)** Report cefinase only. **1st Rx:** ampicillin-clavulanate or SXT or oral expanded- or broad-spectrum cephalosporin or azithromycin **2nd Rx:** ciprofloxacin or imipenem Naturally resistant to penicillin, erythromycin, and clindamycin. Always confirm if resistant to any broad-spectrum cephalosporin or carbapenem.	Perform a cefinase test and report. Most strains that are resistant to ampicillin and amoxicillin produce a TEM-type beta-lactamase. Rare beta-lactamase-negative/ampicillin-resistant strains are resistant to amoxicillin-clavulanate, ampicillin-sulbactam, cefaclor, cefetamet, cefonicid, cefprozil, cefuroxime, and loracarbef despite apparent in vitro susceptible results (21). *Haemophilus* test medium, not Mueller-Hinton-chocolate, is used to do AST on *Haemophilus*; this medium contains NAD, bovine hematin, and yeast extract. **Spot test:** for spinal fluid and respiratory specimens, gram-negative small/coccoid rods, growth on chocolate agar but not BA, or satelliting growth on BA, and a negative rapid porphyrin test identify *H. influenzae* at 95% (20). **Serology:** Encapsulated strains can be serotyped. May request ELISA, agglutination, or immunofluorescence.
Haemophilus parainfluenzae Requires V only.	See *H. influenzae.* Can use ampicillin if beta-lactamase negative.	Do cefinase and report as above. Most are upper respiratory and oral isolates. Can push colony across plate.
Haemophilus paraphrophilus Requires V only.	See *H. influenzae.*	Normal oral flora. Do cefinase and report.

Organism	Antimicrobic information	Extent of identification and comments
Hafnia alvei	K/B, MIC, Etest with enteric criteria. Intrinsic resistance to cephalothin (27). **1st Rx:** imipenem or meropenem **2nd Rx:** ticarcillin-clavulanate or piperacillin-tazobactam or ciprofloxacin Same as for *Enterobacter* spp.	Found in feces of humans and animals (especially birds), sewage, soil, and dairy products (1).
Hantavirus A bunyavirus.	There is no specific treatment or cure for hantavirus infection. Treatment of patients with HPS remains supportive in nature.	HPS is a deadly disease transmitted by infected rodents (deer mouse, cotton and rice rats, and white-footed mouse) through urine, droppings, or saliva. Humans contract the disease when they breathe in aerosolized virus. Not transmitted person-to-person. CDC suggests that a positive serological test result, evidence of viral antigen in tissue by immunohistochemistry, or the presence of amplifiable viral RNA sequences in blood or tissue, with compatible history of HPS, is considered diagnostic for HPS. **Serology:** Detect antigen or RNA in tissue by immunohistochemical methods. Can confirm with IgM antibodies or rising titers of IgG.
Helcococcus kunzii Gram-positive cocci in clusters and tetrads.	MIC value or Etest value.	Vancomycin susceptible, PYR positive, LAP positive, BE positive, NaCl positive. Recovered from intact skin of lower extremities, foot wounds; probably only a colonizer (63).
Helicobacter pylori	CLSI agar dilution method and interpretive criteria for *H. pylori* vs. clarithromycin are available. **1st Rx:** omeprazole + amoxicillin + clarithromycin **2nd Rx:** bismuth + tetracycline + metronidazole + omeprazole	Associated with peptic ulcer disease and cancers of the human GI tract. Gastric, spiral shaped bacteria. Requires 5–10% O_2, 5–12% CO_2, 5–10% H_2. **Serology:** EIAs have sensitivity and specificity of >90% and are better than IFA or CF tests. May grow on selective or nonselective medium at 37°C for 5–7 days. Test of cure: breath test; stool antigen controversial.
Hepatitis viruses	There is no cure for viral hepatitis, and drug therapies exist only for hepatitis C. Doctors recommend rest. There are vaccines available for hepatitis A and B. The hepatitis A vaccine is given to medical workers and travelers. The hepatitis B vaccine is administered to children and high-risk adults.	There are several forms of viral hepatitis, each caused by its own virus. They are the following. Hepatitis A: seen in epidemics and transmitted through fecally contaminated food and water. Serology, IgM anti-HAV and total anti-HAV. Hepatitis B: transmitted by infected blood or blood products, or sexually. HBsAg, HBeAg, anti-HBsAg, anti-HBcAg, and IgM anti-HBeAg are serology markers. Hepatitis C: transmitted by blood from asymptomatic donors and may result in chronic disease. Genotype 1 most common in United States. Serology, anti-HCV and recombinant immunoblot assay. Hepatitis D: occurs in conjunction with hepatitis B and results in either acute or chronic disease. Serology, IgM anti-HDV, anti-HDV, and HDVAg. Hepatitis E: often transmitted by fecally contaminated food in the tropics. Serology, anti-HEV and IgM anti-HEV. Hepatitis disease is either acute (starts and ends quickly) or chronic (long-term progression).

Herpesvirus Includes eight members of the family that can cause human disease: herpes simplex viruses (HSV type 1 [HSV-1] and HSV-2), varicella-zoster virus (VZV, or HSV-3), which causes both chicken pox and shingles, Epstein-Barr virus (EBV, or HSV-4), cytomegalovirus (CMV, or HSV-5), roseola or sixth disease (HSV-6), some roseola and some febrile illness (HSV-7), and Kaposi's sarcoma-associated herpesvirus (KSHV, or HSV-8).	Depending on which member of the herpes family is the etiologic agent; therapy may be selected from acyclovir, ganciclovir, foscarnet, cidofovir, valganciclovir, or in some cases no treatment (39).	Two most common presentations of this virus may be seen as either orofacial lesions or fever blisters (generally HSV-1) or genital lesions (HSV-2). Both produce painful blisters that contain infectious virus. There remains no cure for either. **Serology:** ELISA, immunoblot, CF, and serum neutralization can all test for antibodies with acute and convalescent sera but routine serology cannot distinguish HSV-1 and HSV-2.
Histoplasma One species with two varieties: *H. capsulatum* var. *capsulatum* and *H. capsulatum* var. *duboisii*. The sexual stage is *Ajellomyces capsulatus*.	Submit to reference laboratory for testing. Amphotericin B, itraconazole, and fluconazole are currently useful in treatment of histoplasmosis.	Causes a true systemic mycosis and grows as a mold at 25°C and a yeast at 37°C on brain heart infusion agar with 5% blood. It is endemic in the Tennessee-Ohio-Mississippi river basins. **Serology:** May request double diffusion or compliment fixation tests for antibodies.
HIV See Human immunodeficiency virus		
Hormographiella aspergillata	No data available.	A fungus that is an anamorph of the common inky cap mushroom. Rare cause of pneumonia and endocarditis in humans.
HPIV See Parainfluenza virus		
Human immunodeficiency virus (HIV) HIV-1 is the most frequent cause of AIDS in humans. HIV-2 may cause a milder disease and is primarily found in West Africa.	A variety of antiretroviral therapeutics and regimens are available in addition to therapies and prophylaxis for anticipated infectious diseases.	Laboratory diagnosis requires evaluation of $CD4^+$ T-cell levels in peripheral blood in addition to molecular tests for qualitative and quantitative assays for the virus. **Serology:** Rapid procedures use ELISA effectively. Confirmation by immunoblot analysis for antibodies to gp160/120, gp41, and p24 and p32 antigens (structural proteins). Others may also be found.
***Hymenolepis* spp.** (tapeworms) The genus may contain in excess of 400 species. *H. nana* (referred to as *Vampirolepis nana* by some authors) is a human parasite. *H. diminuta* is less common.	**1st Rx:** praziquantel **2nd Rx:** niclosamide	
Ignavigranum ruoffiae Gram-positive cocci in chains. Named for Kate Ruoff.		Rare from wound and ear abscess (63). Catalase negative, PYR positive, LAP positive, NaCl positive, esculin positive, vancomycin susceptible.

Organism	Antimicrobic information	Extent of identification and comments
Influenza virus H3 and H1 remain common in the United States, but recent emergence of H5N1 in Asia and other parts of the world in avian populations has raised concerns of possible pandemic should human-to-human transmission appear. Influenza A virus has 15 subtypes of HA and 9 subtypes of NA. Influenza A and B viruses have 8 ssRNA segments. Influenza C virus has 7 ssRNA segments, and thogotoviruses have 6 ssRNA segments.	Vaccines usually protect against types A and B but not C. Amantadine, rimantadine, and oseltamivir are therapeutic choices, but resistance to amantadine and rimantadine became common during the 2005–2006 flu season and these drugs are not recommended.	Rapid antigen tests are available to detect types A and B, but recent experience shows a lack of sensitivity and specificity and the results should be interpreted with caution. Influenza A and B viruses cause epidemics of disease almost every winter. In the United States, these seasonal epidemics can cause illness in 10 to 20% of a population and the CDC reports an average of 36,000 deaths and 114,000 hospitalizations per year. Influenza C virus infections cause a mild respiratory illness and are not thought to cause epidemics. A negative rapid antigen test should be followed by culture.
Kawasaki syndrome Occurs at 6 wk to 12 yr of age, with a peak at 1 yr of age (54).	Intravenous immunoglobulin + aspirin.	Unknown cause. Syndrome of increased temperature, rash, conjunctivitis, stomatitis, cervical adenitis, red hands/feet, and coronary artery aneurysms. Some think disease is due to toxin (superantigen) production by staphylococci or streptococci (41).
Kingella denitrificans (f. TM-1, from the fact that it grew on Thayer-Martin agar)	No test method available. Can try MIC value or Etest value if required. No CLSI criteria for testing.	Rare cause of infection. 80% from throat, urinary tract. May confuse with *Neisseria gonorrhoeae* on Thayer-Martin agar, i.e., is glucose positive, maltose negative. Use "Catlin test" to differentiate cocci or coccobacilli from rods: **1.** Inoculate chocolate agar plate with organism using K/B method and add a 10-U penicillin disk. **2.** After growth, sample and Gram stain cells at the edge of the zone of inhibition. **3.** If the cells are rods (*Kingella* or *Moraxella*), they will elongate. **4.** If the cells are true cocci (*Neisseria*), they will remain coccal in shape.
Kingella indologenes	No test method available. Can try MIC value or Etest value if required.	Rarely seen. Confirm identification with another method. Glucose positive, sucrose positive, maltose positive, and indole positive. Similar to *Cardiobacterium hominis.*
Kingella kingae Named for Elizabeth King.	No test method available. Can try MIC value or Etest value if required. Susceptible to penicillin, erythromycin, tetracycline, chloramphenicol, and streptomycin. Combination of penicillin (or ampicillin) plus aminoglycoside reported effective.	Most CDC isolates are from children <5 yr old. Normal in oropharynx. May be difficult to identify on some commercial systems. May pit agar. May look like streptococcus, i.e., coccoid.
Klebsiella oxytoca (Formerly indole-positive *K. pneumoniae*)	K/B, MIC, Etest. Strains of this species can be ESBL producers too. Use *K. pneumoniae* criteria. **1st Rx:** broad-spectrum cephalosporin or fluoroquinolone **2nd Rx:** ticarcillin-clavulanate or ampicillin-sulbactam or piperacillin-tazobactam	

Klebsiella ozaenae Genetically the same as *Klebsiella pneumoniae*; therefore, some call this a subspecies of *K. pneumoniae.*	K/B, MIC, or Etest. **1st Rx:** fluoroquinolones **2nd Rx:** rifampin + SXT	Associated with the tropical disease called ozaena.
Klebsiella pneumoniae Be alert for ESBLs.	K/B, MIC, or Etest. **1st Rx:** broad-spectrum cephalosporin, fluoroquinolone **2nd Rx:** ticarcillin-clavulanate or ampicillin-sulbactam or piperacillin-tazobactam Intrinsic resistance to ampicillin and carbenicillin (27).	Strains that produce ESBLs may be clinically resistant to therapy with penicillins, cephalosporin, or aztreonam despite apparent in vitro susceptibility to some of these agents. *ESBL screening breakpoints are as follows: cefpodoxime (MIC, ≥8 μg/ml), and ceftazidime, aztreonam, cefotaxime, and ceftriaxone would exhibit MIC of ≥2 μg/ml (21).*
Klebsiella rhinoscleromatis Genetically the same as *K. pneumoniae* and often used as a subspecies.	K/B, MIC, or Etest. Same therapy as for *K. ozaenae.*	Associated with the tropical disease called rhinoscleroma.
***Kluyvera* spp.** (f. enteric group 8) New member of the *Enterobacteriaceae* isolated from stool, respiratory, blood, and urine. Environmental organism. Named for A. J. Kluyver.	K/B, MIC, or Etest. Intrinsic resistance to ampicillin (27). Use CLSI enteric charts.	Considered opportunistic pathogens. Now associated with pyelonephritis and soft tissue infections. Four species; *K. ascorbata* and *K. cryocrescens* are common. *K. georgiana* is rare. The fourth is unimportant.
Lacazia loboai (f. *Loboa*) Not yet cultivated.	Although no in vitro data are available, clofazimine has been effective in some cases of lobomycosis.	A yeast-like fungus that causes lobomycosis in humans and dolphins and is mostly tropical. No person-to-person spread.
***Lactobacillus* spp.**	No CLSI criteria available. **1st Rx:** penicillin or ampicillin +/– gentamicin **2nd Rx:** clindamycin, erythromycin Some may be resistant to vancomycin.	Difficult to identify and usually not needed for interpretation. Thirty-four species and 19 groups are known but few are found in humans and they are only rarely pathogenic. May be significant on repeated isolations from sterile sites. Observe long, parallel-sided, thin gram-positive rods; catalase negative.
***Lactococcus* spp.**	No CLSI criteria for interpretation. Resist testing, or use MIC value or Etest value.	Gram-positive coccus in pairs and short chains. Found in urinary tract infections, septicemia, endocarditis (63). Vancomycin susceptible, PYR positive, LAP positive, BE (variable), NaCl positive.
Leclercia adecarboxylata (f. *Escherichia adecarboxylata* and enteric group 41) Named for H. Leclerc.	K/B, MIC, or Etest. Use CLSI enteric charts.	New member of the *Enterobacteriaceae* isolated from respiratory, blood, urine, and wounds. Also found in food and water.
***Legionella* spp.** About 45 species and 60 serogroups (68).	Resist testing or refer to reference lab. **1st Rx:** fluoroquinolone or azithromycin or erythromycin +/– rifampin **2nd Rx:** clarithromycin The most active fluoroquinolones in vitro are trovafloxacin, sparfloxacin, and levofloxacin.	*L. pneumophila* still predominates in humans with 14 serotypes. An aquatic organism found in most natural waters and in man-made cooling facilities. No person-to-person spread. Contracted only from environment. Survives and replicates in free-living amoebae.

Organism	Antimicrobic information	Extent of identification and comments
Leifsonia *L. aquatica* (f. *Corynebacterium aquaticum*) is the only medically relevant species. Named for E. Leifson.		Gram-positive thin rods. Catalase and oxidase positive (diphtheroids are oxidase negative), motile, and oxidize glucose.
Leminorella grimontii (f. enteric group 57) New member of the *Enterobacteriaceae* from feces and occasionally urine. Genus named for Leon Le Minor and his wife, Simone.	K/B, MIC, or Etest. Use CLSI enteric charts.	*L. richardii* is the other species; both produce H_2S. Not much in the literature to document pathogenicity.
***Leptospira* spp.** (50)	No CLSI criteria. **1st Rx:** penicillin G **2nd Rx:** doxycycline Can use oral therapy for less severe cases (66).	Leptospires detected in blood, CSF, and tissues by dark-field or DFA assay. Dark-field is insensitive. DFA is best. Immunohistochemical stains available at CDC. Motile with two subterminal periplasmic flagella and can pass through 0.2-µm filters. Can do direct examination of blood, CSF, and tissue. No antigen tests available. PCR is available but not approved. Organisms isolated in blood (can ship in heparin, oxalate, or citrate) and CSF in the first 10 days after onset, and in urine after 1 wk. PLM-5 or Ellinghausen's medium is used and incubated at room temperature for up to 3 months (usually positive in 2 wk). Antibodies detected after 1 wk of symptoms and peak at 3–4 wk. Using ELISA, a titer of 1:200 is suggestive and 1:800 is strong evidence of disease.
Leptotrichia buccalis	No CLSI criteria. **1st Rx:** penicillin G **2nd Rx:** doxycycline	
***Leuconostoc* spp.**	No CLSI criteria. Refer. **1st Rx:** penicillin or AMP **2nd Rx:** clindamycin, erythromycin, or minocycline Generally resistant to vancomycin.	Vancomycin resistant, PYR negative, LAP negative, BE (variable), NaCl (variable). Gram-positive cocci in chains. May occur in neonates, colonized during delivery.
***Listeria* spp.**	Can do K/B with PEN and AMP disk only. Otherwise report MIC value or Etest value. No CLSI criteria to help. Natural resistance to broad-spectrum cephalosporins and fluoroquinolones. *Do not report cephalosporins as susceptible.* **1st Rx:** ampicillin **2nd Rx:** SXT	Medium to small gram-positive rod; catalase positive; medium colony with small beta-hemolysis. Tumbling motility. Mostly meningitis, encephalitis, septicemia in nonpregnant adults. In pregnancy, a flulike bacteremia can lead to fetal infection and poor birth outcomes. Examples of detection methods from foods: Gene-Trak probe and Listeria-Tek.
Loboa See *Lacazia loboai*		

Lyme disease Caused by *Borrelia burgdorferi.*	No CLSI criteria available. Tick bite: therapy not indicated (64). Early (erythema chronicum migrans): doxycycline or amoxicillin.	At least 24,000 cases reported in the United States in 2002. Transmission occurs in ~10% of bites by infected ticks. Prompt removal of tick decreases risk. Diagnosis is mostly clinical (55). Lab tests support clinical diagnosis but are not the basis for diagnosis or therapy. Test first for antibody by ELISA or fluorescent antibody. If positive, use Western blotting.
Malassezia (f. *Pityrosporum*) Seven species, the most common of which are *M. furfur* (which requires olive oil on medium for growth) and *M. pachydermidis* (which does not require the fatty acids for growth).	MICs in in vitro may be variable, so reference laboratory testing is recommended. Oral ketoconazole or itraconazole are commonly used for treatment of pityriasis versicolor. Antifungal therapy and removal of the catheter are the guidelines for treatment of catheter-related infections. Amphotericin B therapy may be used in these patients with catheter infections.	A lipophilic yeast found superficially on about 90% of humans. Infections are usually from endogenous sources and cause pityriasis versicolor and other skin diseases including white piedra. Occurs especially in patients who are on parenteral nutrition with lipids. Skin scrapings may reveal both hyphae and yeast cells in a "spaghetti and meatball" appearance.
Massilia timonae Some human wound isolates.	Susceptible to most antibiotics, with resistance reported to AMP, cephalothin, and aztreonam (63a).	Motile, aerobic, gram-negative rod, oxidase negative, grows on MacConkey agar, catalase positive, and asaccharolytic. Pale yellow colonies are very tenacious on agar and form flocculation in liquid medium.
Measles virus Causes rubeola, or red measles. A paramyxovirus (ssRNA virus).	Live attenuated vaccine recommended. No specific antiviral therapy.	Causes an acute, contagious disease with prodromal fever, conjunctivitis, coryza, cough, a red blotchy rash, and Koplik spots on the buccal mucosa. Extremely communicable from slightly before the prodromal period to 4 days after appearance of rash; minimal after second day of rash. About 1 child in every 1,000 who get measles will develop encephalitis. **Serology:** IgM can be demonstrated at the time of the rash but serology is more for immune status and not for clinical diagnosis.
Metapneumovirus Causes an emerging infectious disease.	No specific therapy. Symptoms are usually treated.	Human metapneumovirus, an ssRNA virus first isolated in 2001 from hospitalized children in The Netherlands, is a paramyxovirus that causes acute respiratory tract infections. Most children are seropositive by 5 yr of age. It is genetically most similar to the avian pneumovirus, hence its name.
Methylobacterium mesophilicum (f. *Pseudomonas mesophilica*, *Vibrio extorquens*, and *Corynebacterium rubrum*)	Do not test. No CLSI criteria. Refer if required. Do conventional MIC at 30°C at 48 h, and report values only.	Oxidase-positive; urea-positive; nonfermenting gram-negative rods. Can use Biolog or MIDI system for identification. Slow growing; produces a pink pigment. An environmental isolate. May contaminate stored agar plates. May cause septicemia, continuous ambulatory peritoneal dialysis-related peritonitis, nosocomial problems. Poorly staining, amorphous with many nonstaining vacuoles.
***Microbacterium* spp.**	See Diphtheroids. Usually susceptible to vancomycin. Other drugs are unpredictable and must be tested on significant isolates. Report MIC only.	Microbacteria account for most all yellow-pigmented coryneform bacteria isolated from humans (colors from pale yellow to orange). Too difficult to identify to species level.

Organism	Antimicrobic information	Extent of identification and comments
Micrococcus spp. (6)	K/B, MIC, Etest. Use staphylococcal interpretive criteria.	Usually saprophytic; occasionally opportunistic. *M. luteus* and *M. varians* are yellow pigmented and are the human isolates. *M. roseus* is pink. *M. luteus* is nonpigmented. (Bacitracin / Furazolidone) *Micrococcus*: S / R *Staphylococcus*: R / S
Microsporum Consists of 17 species. Commonly isolated species include *M. audouinii* (anthropophilic), *M. gallinae* (zoophilic [birds]), *M. ferrugineum* (anthropophilic), *M. distortum*, *M. nanum* (geophilic and zoophilic [swine]), *M. canis* (zoophilic [cats and dogs]), *M. gypseum* (geophilic), *M. cookei* (geophilic and from animal fur), and *M. vanbreuseghemii.*	Oral terbinafine and itraconazole are used for treatment of *Microsporum* infections.	One of the three genera that cause dermatophycosis mostly affecting hair and skin, and, only rarely, nails. Spindle-shaped macroconidia are characteristic.
Moellerella wisconsensis (f. enteric group 46) New member of the *Enterobacteriaceae* isolated from feces and water; unknown pathogenicity. Genus named for Vagn Moeller.	K/B, MIC, Etest. Use CLSI enteric charts.	Biochemically inactive. Colonies resemble *E. coli* on MacConkey and eosin methylene blue agar. Six of the first nine strains received at CDC were from Wisconsin.
Moraxella catarrhalis (f. *Branhamella catarrhalis*)	Resist testing if possible. Otherwise, use Etest and report value only or refer to reference lab. >95% are cefinase positive (BD Biosciences). **1st Rx:** ampicillin-clavulanate or oral expanded- and broad-spectrum cephalosporin or SXT. Use ampicillin for beta-lactamase-negative strains. **2nd Rx:** azithromycin, clarithromycin, or dirithromycin Naturally resistant to trimethoprim. Always confirm if resistant to ciprofloxacin.	Spot test: gram-negative diplococci, oxidase positive, grow on BA and chocolate agar, and positive rapid butyrate esterase or positive rapid DNase test identifies *M. catarrhalis* at 95% (20).
***Moraxella* spp.**	Resist testing if possible. Otherwise, use Etest and report value only or refer to reference lab.	Do cefinase only. All are gram-negative rods and catalase positive (except *M. bovis*). May need help to distinguish coccobacilli from true cocci, so use the "Catlin" test described above for *Kingella*.
Moraxella atlantae (f. M-3)		Grows poorly with a small, spreading colony. May corrode agar. Isolates from blood, CSF, spleen but very rare. Do cefinase only.
Moraxella lacunata (f. *Moraxella liquefaciens*)		Needs serum even for slow growth. May take 2 wk. Eye isolates, but rare today. Pits agar. See plump gram-negative rods in pairs and chains. Large dark zones may appear on chocolate agar. Strongly catalase positive. Do cefinase only.

Moraxella nonliquefaciens		The most common *Moraxella* sp. in the urinary tract. Common in nose. Probably nonpathogenic. More fastidious than other *Moraxella* spp. except for *M. lacunata.* Do cefinase only.
Moraxella osloensis (f. *Moraxella* [*Mima*] *polymorpha*)	See *Moraxella* spp. above	Small, alpha-hemolytic colonies that grow well without enrichment. Isolated from blood, CSF, urinary tract infections. Rapid urea positive. Do cefinase only.
Morganella morganii **(or *Morganella* spp.)** (f. *Proteus morganii*) Two subspecies of *M. morganii*: subsp. *morganii* and subsp. *sibonii*	K/B, MIC, Etest. Intrinsic resistance to polymyxins, ampicillin, and cephalothin. **1st Rx:** imipenem or meropenem or broad-spectrum cephalosporin or fluoroquinolone **2nd Rx:** aztreonam, or any beta-lactam + inhibitor.	Etiology is doubtful. Found in urine, sputum, feces, wounds.
Mucor Common species are *M. amphibiorum, M. circinelloides, M. hiemalis, M. indicus, M. racemosus,* and *M. ramosissimus.*	Few data available to support a therapeutic model but amphotericin B is the most commonly used antifungal agent. Submit to reference lab for testing. Response rates are often unsatisfactory.	Naturally occurring in nature and often seen as laboratory contaminants, but can cause human infection (zygomycosis). Usually unable to grow at 37°C, but occasional strains are thermotolerant and are the ones isolated from humans. Produces wide, practically nonseptate hyphae.
Mucormycosis See Zygomycetes		
Mumps virus A paramyxovirus.	According to CDC, one dose of mumps vaccine prevents about 80% of mumps and two doses prevent about 90% of cases. No virus-specific therapy is available.	In the United States, since 2001, an average of 265 mumps cases (range, 231–293) have been reported each year. Large outbreaks may occur, as in 2005, when early cases were reported in Iowa. Symptoms are fever, headache, muscle aches, tiredness, and loss of appetite followed by onset of parotitis. One in five older males may experience swollen testicles. Lifelong immunity occurs after infection. **Serology:** Not needed for diagnosis. A fourfold rise in antibody titer can be demonstrated in infection and there is only one serotype.
Mycobacterium avium **complex (MAC)** Consists of *M. avium* and *M. intracellulare.* A new MAC-X strain may be added as a new species, which is probe positive for MAC but probe negative for *M. avium* or *M. intracellulare.*	Most are multiply resistant, and we should resist sending them out unless we have ID consult approval. **1st Rx:** clarithromycin or azithromycin + ethambutol + rifampin, and others can be added if necessary Regimen for HIV patients should have clarithromycin or azithromycin for life.	MAC is ubiquitous in nature and environmental sources. Low pathogenicity and single positive specimens with low numbers are occasionally found in persons without apparent disease. Causes four patterns of disease: solitary nodules, nodular bronchiectasis, TB-like infiltrates and diffuse infiltrates in immunocompromised. Is the leading cause of localized mycobacterial lymphadenitis in 1- to 5-yr-old children. HIV-negative individuals usually have pulmonary infection.

Organism	Antimicrobic information	Extent of identification and comments
***Mycobacterium fortuitum* complex** Consists of *M. abscessus*, *M. chelonae*, *M. fortuitum* group, *M. mucogenicum*, and *M. genavense*.	These members differ in their drug susceptibilities and in the type of infections they cause. Refer for testing.	*M. abscessus* causes 90% of chronic lung disease due to rapidly growing species and 90% of post-tympanostomy tube otitis media. *M. chelonae*: slowest growing of this group, requiring 28–30°C. Most likely of the group to be encountered in immunosuppressed patients. (Clarithromycin is first-choice antimicrobial.) *M. fortuitum*: most common species in the group associated with nosocomial outbreaks or pseudo-outbreaks. *M. mucogenicum*: mucoid and from tap water. Often recovered from a single sample of sputum which is not clinically significant. Can cause disease, however. *M. genavense*: slow growing, causes disease in psittacine birds. Found in AIDS patients. Needs 6–8 wk to grow.
***Mycobacterium tuberculosis* complex** Consists of *M. tuberculosis*, *M. bovis* (causes TB in humans, cattle, primates and some birds), *M. microti* (causes TB in voles and local lesions in guinea pigs, not humans), *M. africanum* (causes TB in tropical Africa, probably should not be a separate species). Carried on airborne nuclei 1–5 μm in size.	Follow special procedure or refer. Some labs use rifampin resistance as a marker to predict resistance to other TB drugs. If the organism is susceptible to rifampin, the patient outcome is usually okay even if the organism is resistant to isoniazid or streptomycin (M. Salfinger, personal communication). Multiple therapy options depending on prevalence of resistance and results of testing. Always use multiple drug combinations.	High prevalence population: underserved ethnic minorities, homeless, prison inmates, alcoholics, drug users, the elderly, and foreign-born persons from areas of endemicity. High rate of progression from latent to active disease: those with underlying conditions, people infected <2 yr, children <4 yr old, and persons with positive X ray. HIV is the greatest risk factor for progression. Latent infection: 10% risk over lifetime for progression. HIV positive: 10–15% risk per year for progression. **Serology:** Skin test is widest used immunology test. *Mycobacterium bovis* BCG vaccination gives positive skin test but not long-lasting immunity.
Mycobacterium **(other species)**	Refer as requested. Confirm with infectious disease consult if possible.	*M. simiae*: in southwestern United States. Found in tap water. Clinical disease similar to MAC disease. *M. szulgai*: rare in humans. *M. ulcerans*: ulcers on lower extremities; in tropics. *M. xenopi*: pulmonary disease with an underlying disease somewhere. *M. kansasii*: photochromogen. Causes chronic disease resembling TB. *M. malmoense*: rare in United States, more common in northern Europe. Usually in young children with cervical lymphadenitis or in adults with chronic disease. *M. marinum*: mostly cutaneous "fish tank granuloma." *M. gordonae*: commonly encountered and usually nonpathogenic. Only one clinically significant isolate in the literature.
Mycoplasma hominis	No test necessary. **1st Rx:** doxycycline **2nd Rx:** clindamycin Resistant to erythromycin and rifampin; tetracycline resistance emerging.	Primarily isolated from urogenital sites. Found in sexually active adults along with the more common *Ureaplasma urealyticum*. Microscopy not useful and antigen tests are not commercially available. PCR amplification tests have been developed but are less helpful than culture. Do not use cotton swabs. Can be recovered on SP4 glucose broth and agar supplemented with arginine. Culture positive in 2–5 days.

Mycoplasma pneumoniae	No test necessary. Beta-lactams not useful. **1st Rx:** erythromycin, azithromycin, clarithromycin, or fluoroquinolone **2nd Rx:** doxycycline	Causes about 20% of community acquired pneumonia and up to 50% in some groups. Causes illness in children, adolescents, and young adults. Microscopy not useful. Several antigen tests are commercially available but are insensitive. PCR amplification tests have been developed. Do not use cotton swabs. Can be recovered on SP4 glucose broth and agar. Culture positive in 3 wk or more.
Myroides odoratus (f. *Flavobacterium odoratum*)	See *Flavobacterium odoratum*	
Neisseria cinerea	Etest or refer.	Plump cocci in pairs or clusters. Small gray-white colonies. Normal in nasopharynx.
Neisseria elongata subsp. *nitroreducens* (f. *Moraxella* M-6; CDC M-6)	Etest or refer.	Associated with endocarditis. Catalase negative.
Neisseria flavescens	Etest or refer. No CLSI criteria available for testing.	Yellow pigment on Loeffler's agar. Rare in humans but has come from blood and CSF. Does not grow on TM.
Neisseria gonorrhoeae The cause of the second most commonly reported disease in the United States, second only to *Chlamydia trachomatis*. SPS is inhibitory (70).	Special procedures are available using special medium (21). Can also do Etest if necessary. Usually susceptible to broad-spectrum cephalosporin. Beta-lactamase test cannot detect chromosomally mediated resistance; must do disk diffusion or agar dilution method. May not be useful since PEN, AMP, or amoxicillin is not a drug of choice anyway. **1st Rx:** ceftriaxone or cefpodoxime or cefixime **2nd Rx:** ofloxacin and other fluoroquinolones Always confirm if resistant to any broad-spectrum cephalosporin. Sexual partners should be treated.	Always best to test for presence of *Chlamydia* along with *N. gonorrhoeae*. If *N. gonorrhoeae* positive, treat for both gonorrhea and *Chlamydia* infection. Grows on Thayer-Martin agar, as do *N. meningitidis* and *N. lactamica*. Other neisseriae do not. Eighty-five percent of all sexually transmitted disease occurs in persons aged 15–30 yr. **1.** The presence of urethritis in HIV-positive males increases the amount of HIV in their semen, thus increasing likelihood of HIV transmission. **2.** The presence of urethritis in persons who are HIV negative increases the likelihood of acquiring HIV (indicates promiscuous relationships) (16). **Serology:** Antibody detection not very useful. EIAs are effective but Gram stain, culture, and/or nucleic acid probes are most useful.
Neisseria lactamica	Etest or refer.	Normal in nasopharynx of infants and children. Rarely pathogenic. Not much data.
Neisseria meningitidis SPS is inhibitory. Work carefully with this organism. It can easily cause laboratory-acquired infections.	Use CLSI special MIC test or just report value from Etest. *Do not do a K/B*, since the in vitro disk tests are unreliable. **1st Rx:** penicillin **2nd Rx:** ceftriaxone, cefuroxime, cefotaxime Always confirm if resistant to high-level penicillin or to ciprofloxacin. Use prophylaxis for close contacts of meningitis patients with rifampin, ceftriaxone, or ciprofloxacin.	Grows on TM. This organism is genetically the same as *N. gonorrhoeae*. May see tetrads in young cultures because of the way the cells divide. Normal in human nasopharynx. **Serology:** Direct antigen tests of CSF not recommended. Patients deficient in complement components C5, C6, C7, and C8 more prone to disseminated disease. Antigen tests detect serogroups A, B, C, Y, and W1135.

Organism	Antimicrobic information	Extent of identification and comments
Neisseria mucosa	Etest or refer.	Common in nasopharynx. Mucoid, adherent colony. May cause pneumonia. Does not grow on TM.
Neisseria sicca	Etest or refer.	Dry, wrinkled, adherent colony. Does not grow on TM.
Neisseria subflava	Etest or refer.	Smooth colony that autoagglutinates in saline. Also yellow pigmented on Loeffler's agar. Does not grow on TM.
Neisseria weaveri (f. *Moraxella* sp. strain M-5; CDC M-6)		Clinical isolates associated with dog bites.
Nematodes (roundworms, helminths) *Ancylostoma duodenale* (hookworm) *Ascaris lumbricoides* (ascariasis) *Brugia malayi* (filariasis) *Brugia timori* (filariasis) *Dracunculus medinensis* (guinea worm) *Enterobius vermicularis* (pinworm) *Loa loa* (loiasis) *Necatur americanus* (hookworm) *Onchocerca volvulus* (river blindness) *Strongyloides stercoralis* *Toxocara canis* (larva migrans) *Trichinella spiralis* (trichinosis) *Trichostrongylus orientalis* *Trichuris trichiura* (whipworm) *Wuchereria bancrofti* (filariasis)	The phylum Nematoda contains more than 500,000 species, only a few of which cause infections in humans usually accompanied by eosinophilia and elevated IgE levels. **Rx:** Various therapeutic options exist, depending on the organism and the body site infected. Options include ivermectin, albendazole, mebendazole, pyrantel pamoate, metronidazole, and diethylcarbamazine.	
Nocardia spp. Aerobic actinomycetes. Genus contains 22 species, 13 of which are clinically important. Form extensive branched hyphae that fragment into rod-shaped to coccoid, nonmotile elements and usually form aerial hyphae that may be seen only microscopically.	No CLSI criteria. *N. asteroides* and *N. brasiliensis*: **1st Rx:** SXT; high-dose sulfonamides **2nd Rx:** minocycline (*N. asteroides*), ampicillin-clavulanate (*N. brasiliensis*) (resistant to imipenem)	*N. asteroides* found primarily in the Southeast and Southwest. Most are soil saprophytes. Infection usually by inhalation. Prolonged therapy often required. *N. brasiliensis* mostly in tropical countries and causes primary cutaneous infections. Resistant to imipenem.

***Nocardiopsis* spp.** Two of seven species have been isolated from humans: *N. dassonvillei* (the only species of interest in humans) and *N. synnemataformans.*	No CLSI criteria. Refer to reference laboratory for testing. **1st Rx:** SXT (33)	Not acid fast; susceptible to lysozyme; urea positive, nitrate positive. Observe branching with internal spores. Coarsely wrinkled colony and folded with good aerial mycelium. Substrate hyphae are yellow, orange-brown for *N. dassonvillei*, and deep pimiento for *N. synnemataformans.* Causes white-grain mycetoma.
Noroviruses (Norwalk-like viruses) Genus *Norovirus*, family *Caliciviridae*, is a group of related, single-stranded RNA, nonenveloped viruses that cause acute gastroenteritis in humans. *Norovirus* was recently approved as the official genus name for the group of viruses provisionally described as "Norwalk-like viruses" (NLV).	No specific therapy is available for viral gastroenteritis.	Noroviruses are named after the original strain "Norwalk virus," which caused an outbreak of gastroenteritis in a school in Norwalk, Ohio, in 1968. CDC data suggest the incubation period for norovirus-associated gastroenteritis in humans is usually between 24 and 48 h (median in outbreaks, 33–36 h), but cases can occur within 12 h of exposure. Common on cruise ships. Norovirus infection usually presents as acute-onset vomiting, watery nonbloody diarrhea with abdominal cramps, and nausea. Low-grade fever also occasionally occurs, and vomiting is more common in children than in adults.
Obesumbacterium proteus New member of the *Enterobacteriaceae* found in breweries, not in humans.	Do not test.	Not a human pathogen.
Ochrobactrum anthropi (f. Vd-1; Vd-2)	MIC value or Etest value only. Resistant to carbenicillin. Susceptible to gentamicin. No CLSI criteria for interpretation.	Similar biochemically to *Agrobacterium*. Not sure of its pathogenicity. Isolates from blood, urine, wound, stool, water. Gram-negative, motile rod; urea positive overnight.
Oerskovia turbata	See Diphtheroids.	Normal inhabitant of soil. Not usually a pathogen. Smells like dirt and is yellow pigmented. Colonies penetrate the agar. Some corynebacterium identification systems identify this isolate well.
Oligella ureolytica (f. IVe)	Refer. No CLSI criteria for interpretation.	Gram-negative short rod, motile with very long flagella. Catalase positive, oxidase positive, urea positive instantly. Often from male urine specimens associated with stones. May be confused with *Brucella*, which does not come from urine. If you have a urine isolate that is inert and strongly urea positive quickly, think of *Oligella.*
Oligella urethralis (f. *Moraxella urethralis*, M-4)	Refer. You can try an Etest, but report value only. Susceptible to penicillin. No CLSI criteria.	Mostly from urinary tract of women.
Opisthorchis See Trematodes		
Orientia tsutsugamushi Causes scrub typhus. See *Rickettsia*		Spread by *Leptotrombidium* (chigger) bite.
Paecilomyces Several species, but the most common are *P. lilacinus* and *P. variotii.*	Limited data available for susceptibility interpretations. Submit to reference laboratory for testing. Amphotericin B in combination with flucytosine has been successfully used for *P. lilacinus.*	Normal environmental fungus that is usually considered a contaminant but has been isolated from humans from infection of skin and of many organs.

Organism	Antimicrobic information	Extent of identification and comments
Pandoraea spp.	Refer or report MIC value only.	Biochemically similar to *Burkholderia* and *Ralstonia*. Differentiated by fatty acid profiles.
Panic values (critical values) (26, 43, 47) This first tier of calling should be limited to results that represent a truly life-threatening event, or that need immediate attention therapeutically or epidemiologically. A second-tier calling of significant results, i.e., agents reportable to federal or state agencies, is an option, as are courtesy calls requested by specific physicians. Infection control may require some results to be called. (Watch out! You can spend too much time calling results that have little impact on patient care.)	No universal standardized list is available, and the local facility usually develops its own. Use common sense for good patient outcomes. Panic values should be telephoned to the patient's physician or the physician designee. Results to be reported by telephone may include the following: AFB or fluorescent smear positive for *M. tuberculosis* Blood culture or blood product (preinfusion) positive and smear positive Cryptococcal antigen positive (latex or India ink) CSF smear and culture positive Malaria smear positive STAT request results Select agents confirmed by reference laboratory (anthrax, tularemia, plague, etc.) Sterile fluid culture positive Streptococcus, group B from newborn Viral DFA or culture positives for herpes simplex virus (HSV) from CSF and blood, respiratory syncytial virus/influenza virus, cytomegalovirus, varicella-zoster virus or HSV from immunosuppressed patients. Some labs prefer to call most positive viral tests.	
Pantoea agglomerans (f. *Enterobacter agglomerans*)	K/B, MIC, Etest. Use CLSI enteric criteria for AST.	From a group of plant pathogens now belonging to the genus *Erwinia*. Some isolates have been from humans. The other species, *P. dispersa*, is not a human isolate. May produce yellow pigment.
Paracoccidioides brasiliensis The only species in this genus.	Susceptibility data are limited. Submit to reference laboratory for testing if required. Amphotericin B, sulfonamides, and ketoconazole have been used for treatment. Itraconazole is now the drug of choice.	A thermally dimorphic fungus found mostly in Central and South America and which causes South American blastomycosis, a chronic granulomatous disease that spreads from lungs to nasal mucosa and the mouth. The disease may take months to express. May disseminate further. **Serology:** May request complement fixation and immunoassay tests. Skin testing used for epidemiology but is negative in acute cases.
Paragonimus See Trematodes		
Parainfluenza virus Most common serotypes of human parainfluenza viruses (HPIV): HPIV-1, HPIV-2, and HPIV-3. HPIV-4 (with two subtypes) is much less common. These are negative-sense ssRNA viruses.	No vaccine is currently available.	According to CDC, human parainfluenza viruses are second to RSV as a common cause of lower respiratory tract disease in young children. Like RSV, these viruses can cause repeated infections throughout life, usually manifested by an upper respiratory tract illness (e.g., a cold and/or sore throat) and spread early in the disease. More serious disease can occur. The most distinctive clinical feature of HPIV-1 and HPIV-2 is croup (i.e., laryngotracheobronchitis); HPIV-3 is more often associated with bronchiolitis and pneumonia.
Pasteurella aerogenes	Rare from humans. Four of eight cases have been from swine bites. If this is the answer you got from your identification system, it is probably wrong. Check it out.	
Pasteurella haemolytica	No CLSI interpretive criteria available. Refer or try Etest and report value only.	The only beta-hemolytic pasteurella, but hemolysis may be lost on subculture. Mostly animal sources; low potential to cause human illness. No CLSI criteria.

Pasteurella multocida	No CLSI interpretive criteria available. Resist testing and refer if possible; or do MIC value or Etest value. **1st Rx:** penicillin G or ampicillin or amoxicillin **2nd Rx:** doxycycline, ampicillin-clavulanate, SXT, or expanded-spectrum cephalosporins	Tiny, nonmotile, gram-negative rods. Catalase positive, oxidase positive, does not grow on MacConkey agar. Normal in dogs and cats. Common in humans but not transmitted person-to-person. May show multiple colony types from pure culture.
Pasteurella pneumotropica	Do not test.	No human isolates.
Pasteurella ureae See *Actinobacillus ureae*	Refer if required.	
Pediococcus acidilactici The only species in its genus.	No CLSI interpretive criteria available. Etest or refer.	Gram-positive cocci in clusters and tetrads. No clearly defined syndrome in humans. Probably not significant except from sterile sites in severely compromised patients. Vancomycin resistant, PYR negative, LAP positive, BE positive, NaCl (variable).
Penicillium Many species, but the most common are *P. chrysogenum*, *P. citrinum*, *P. janthinellum*, *P. marneffei*, and *P. purpurogenum*.	Submit to reference laboratory for testing. Amphotericin B, oral itraconazole, and oral fluconazole have been used in treatment of *P. marneffei*.	With only one exception (*Penicillium marneffei*, which is thermally dimorphic), the *Penicillium* spp. are filamentous fungi. Most are contaminants, but *P. marneffei* is considered pathogenic. Any of the species may be opportunistic in humans. *P. marneffei* particularly causes disease in AIDS patients in Southeast Asia and in patients with malignancies.
Phaeoannellomyces werneckii (f. *Exophiala werneckii*)	Submit to reference laboratory for susceptibility testing.	Causes tinea nigra, which is irregularly shaped brown to black spots on the palm of the hands or occasionally on other parts of the body.
Phaeohyphomycosis Cutaneous, subcutaneous, or systemic infection caused by dematiaceous fungi which may include *Scedosporium*, *Bipolaris*, *Wangiella*, *Curvularia*, *Exophiala*, *Alternaria*, and others.		
Phialophora Eight species: *P. americana*, *P. bubakii*, *P. europaea*, *P. parasitica*, *P. reptans*, *P. repens*, *P. richardsiae*, and *P. verrucosa*.	Submit to reference lab for testing since MICs may vary. Amphotericin B, itraconazole, voriconazole, and terbinafine have been successfully used in some cases.	A dematiaceous, filamentous fungus, common in nature, that can cause human infections. *P. verrucosa* commonly causes chromoblastomycosis and in tissue appears as dark, round, septate cells.
Piedraia *P. hortae* and *P. quintanilhae* are the two species in this genus.	Limited MIC data available for treatment of black piedra. Approaches include shaving of affected hair, topical salicylic acid, formaldehyde, oral ketoconazole, or azole creams, but relapses are common.	A dematiaceous fungus. *P. hortae* causes black piedra, a disease with small, stony, hard, dark nodules along hair shafts, in humans. White piedra is caused by *Trichosporon beigelii*. *P. quintanilhae* is found in chimpanzees in Central Africa.
Plesiomonas shigelloides (see lysine/arginine/ornithine table below)	No CLSI criteria. If required, do MIC value or Etest value only. Best idea is to refer for testing. **1st Rx:** ciprofloxacin **2nd Rx:** SXT	May agglutinate in *Shigella* group D antisera. Not normal in humans and may cause diarrhea. Oxidase positive. Usually self-limited and may not require therapy.

	Lysine	Arginine	Ornithine
Plesiomonas	+	+	+
Aeromonas	−	+	−

(17% of *Aeromonas* isolates are lysine positive)

Organism	Antimicrobic information	Extent of identification and comments
***Pneumocystis jiroveci* (*P. carinii*)** A yeastlike fungal microorganism. Jiroveci is pronounced "yee row vet see." The taxonomy remains unresolved, but *P. jiroveci* appears to be the human-associated isolate. *P. carinii* is actually found in nonhuman hosts. Other species exist.	**1st Rx:** SXT Others include dapsone, pentamidine, and atovaquone.	*Pneumocystis* pneumonia (PCP or pneumocystitis) is the most common opportunistic infection in people with HIV; without treatment, nearly 85% of people with HIV would eventually develop it. Does not stain well with periodic acid-Schiff stain. Calcofluor white is good at distinguishing the coffee bean-shaped intracystic bodies (*Cryptococcus* does not have these bodies).
Poliovirus An enterovirus; a member of the picornaviruses ("pico" = tiny; "rna" = RNA; thus, a picornavirus).	Both heat-killed and attenuated vaccines are available and very effective.	Replicate in oropharynx or intestine, then results in a viremia. Disease ranges from subclinical to paralytic. **Serology:** Diagnosis based on viral neutralization in culture.
Pragia fontium New member of the *Enterobacteriaceae* found in water and feces.	K/B, MIC, or Etest. Use CLSI enteric criteria, but no evidence of pathogenicity.	H_2S-positive enteric bacterium. Similar to *Budvicia*.
Prion diseases A prion is an abnormal, transmissible agent that can induce abnormal folding of normal cellular prion proteins in the brain. Long incubation period. Rapidly progressive and always fatal.	No therapy available.	Human diseases: Creutzfeldt-Jakob disease, Gerstmann-Sträussler-Scheinker syndrome, fatal familial insomnia, and kuru. Animal diseases: bovine spongiform encephalophathy, chronic wasting disease, scrapie, transmissible mink encephalopathy, feline spongiform encephalopathy, and ungulate spongiform encephalophathy.
Proteus mirabilis	K/B, MIC, or Etest. Use CLSI enteric criteria. If the organism is tetracycline susceptible, then it likely is not a *Proteus* sp. **1st Rx:** ampicillin **2nd Rx:** SXT	*Proteus* is the only organism we isolate that swarms and stinks! Do a spot indole test (negative) and sign it out.
Proteus penneri (f. indole-negative *P. vulgaris*)	Use CLSI enteric criteria. Also intrinsically resistant to tetracycline. All *P. penneri* and some *P. mirabilis* strains are ampicillin resistant (20).	
Proteus vulgaris	Use CLSI enteric criteria. Also, intrinsically resistant to polymyxins, tetracycline, ampicillin, and nitrofurantoin (27). **1st Rx:** broad-spectrum cephalosporins or fluoroquinolones **2nd Rx:** antipseudomonal aminoglycoside	

Protozoa (common ones considered pathogenic) (37) About 50,000 species, with about half being parasitic.	*Trichomonas vaginalis* is a flagellate that is found worldwide. Males carry the infection but are usually asymptomatic. The organism feeds on bacteria and white blood cells and can live in bath water, on toilet seats, or on washcloths. Diagnosis is by finding the parasite in discharges or by culture. The drug of choice is metronidazole. *Trypanosoma rhodesiense* or *T. gambiense* causes African sleeping sickness and are transmitted by the tsetse fly. When the central nervous system becomes involved, the classic symptoms of sleeping sickness are induced. Chagas' disease is common in Mexico and South America and is caused by *T. cruzi. Leishmania donovani* causes leishmaniasis and is transmitted by sand flies. Treatment consists of antimonial compounds. *Giardia lamblia* is described above. *Entamoeba histolytica* causes amoebic dysentery (often called "Montezuma's revenge" by travelers). Several antibiotics are used, including metronidazole (the drug of choice), tetracycline, and chloroquine. *Naegleria fowleri* causes amoebic meningoencephalitis and is normally a free-living amoeba, as is *Acanthamoeba*, which is dangerous for contact lens wearers. It colonizes the nasal epithelium and then travels down nerve tracts to the brain. *Balantidium coli* causes balantidiasis, which is a form of dysentery; it is the only ciliated protozoan parasite of humans. *Toxoplasma gondii* causes toxoplasmosis as a result of ingestion of infective cysts of the parasite. In congenital toxoplasmosis, a mother infected at the time of conception or during pregnancy transmits the infection to the developing fetus. The parasite infects the fetus by crossing the placental barrier. *Cryptosporidium parvum* causes cryptosporidiosis. The infectious dose is thought to be less than 10 organisms, and presumably 1 organism can initiate an infection. Watery diarrhea, cramps, and headache are common. Malaria, the world's most prevalent vector-borne disease, is caused by the *Plasmodium* species and has been known since the time of the ancient Egyptians. One thousand cases of malaria are reported annually in the United States, while 500 million people are infected worldwide each year and 2 million–3 million die.	
Providencia alcalifaciens Rare in humans. Be suspicious of the identification result. ***Providencia rettgeri*** ***Providencia stuartii***	K/B, MIC, or Etest. **1st Rx:** amikacin or broad-spectrum cephalosporin or fluoroquinolone **2nd Rx:** SXT	Intrinsic resistance to polymyxins, nitrofurantoin, cephalothin, and tetracycline (27).
***Providencia stuartii*, urea positive**	Use CLSI criteria for routine susceptibility.	
Pseudallescheria boydii (f. *Allescheria* and *Petriellidium*) The only species in the genus and the sexual state of *Scedosporium apiospermum*.	Submit to reference laboratory for testing. Often resistant to amphotericin B. Ketoconazole, itraconazole, and voriconazole may be successful.	Normal in nature but can be an opportunistic pathogen in mostly immunosuppressed hosts. One of the causes of white-grain mycetoma. Almost any organ can be involved, including the central nervous system (which can be involved in near-drowning victims).
Pseudomonas aeruginosa	K/B, MIC, or Etest. Resistance to beta-lactams may arise during therapy. Very rare to see gentamicin, tobramycin, and amikacin resistance concurrently. **1st Rx:** antipseudomonal penicillin, imipenem, tobramycin, ciprofloxacin, ticarcillin-clavulanate, piperacillin-tazobactam, or aztreonam **2nd Rx:** for serious infections: (antipseudomonal penicillins or broad-spectrum cephalosporins, or aztreonam, or ticarcillin-clavulanate or piperacillin-tazobactam or imipenem) + (meropenem or tobramycin or ciprofloxacin)	Spot tests are acceptable to identify this organism, although AST is necessary. Very mucoid strains have poor biochemical reactions. Oxidase positive, typical smell, and colony morphology (blue-green pigment) are 95% diagnostic! (Rare *Aeromonas* isolates can have similar colonies but no odor. *Aeromonas* is indole positive, and *Pseudomonas* is indole negative.) No biochemicals needed. In normal patient populations, if isolated in stool as >3+, do AST and report; otherwise, do not report.
Pseudomonas fluorescens, P. putida*, and *P. mendocina	K/B, MIC, Etest. Instruments will report as "fluorescens/putida group."	None of these have blue-green pigment. *P. aeruginosa*, *P. fluorescens*, and *P. putida* are called the "fluorescent pseudomonads." *P. mendocina* can be confused with nonpigmented *P. aeruginosa*. *P. fluorescens* and *P. putida* are rare in clinical specimens, and both grow best at 25°C.

Organism	Antimicrobic information	Extent of identification and comments
Pseudomonas mallei Causes glanders. ***Pseudomonas pseudomallei*** Causes melioidosis.	***P. mallei* Rx:** sulfadiazine, SXT ***P. pseudomallei* Rx:** ceftazidime or amoxicillin-clavulanate, SXT	Not normally found in the United States. Do not attempt to work up from suspected patients. Submit to an LRN reference laboratory. Resistance to SXT appearing in Southeast Asia (66).
Pseudomonas oryzihabitans (f. *Flavimonas oryzihabitans*, Ve-2) The *Flavimonas* name is replaced by *Pseudomonas* (3).	MIC value or Etest value only. Disk test unreliable.	Yellow pigmented but oxidase negative. Wrinkled colony. Similar to *Chryseomonas luteola*. Associated with septicemia and prosthetic valve endocarditis. Esculin negative.
Pseudomonas paucimobilis (f. IIk-1)	Do not test. If necessary, try Etest. No CLSI criteria. Do MIC and report value only.	Weakly motile. Bright yellow pigment. Sometimes seen with respiratory equipment.
Pseudomonas pickettii (f. Va-2) See *Ralstonia pickettii*	No CLSI interpretive criteria. Refer or try Etest value.	
Pseudomonas putrefaciens See *Shewanella putrefaciens*	No CLSI interpretive criteria. Refer or try Etest value.	
Pseudomonas stutzeri (f. Vb-1)	No CLSI interpretive criteria. Refer or try Etest value.	Wrinkled colony (lactose negative) like *P. pseudomallei* (lactose positive). Colonies are adherent on primary isolation but later become smooth. Mainly comes from soil and water. May have a slight yellow pigment.
Psychrobacter phenylpyruvicus (f. *Moraxella phenylpyruvica*; CDC M-2) Some within this group will likely be changed to *Rhodobacter massiliensis* and a possible new genus, *Haematobacter* (proposed) (41a).	No CLSI criteria.	Phenylalanine deaminase positive; grows at 40°C; tolerates NaCl up to 9%.
Rahnella aquatilis New member of the *Enterobacteriaceae* found in water; not pathogenic for humans.	No need to test unless from sterile site. Then, use K/B, MIC, or Etest.	Rare human infections have been in immunocompromised persons (1).
Ralstonia pickettii (f. *Burkholderia pickettii*, *Pseudomonas pickettii*, CDC Va-1, Va-2) *R. pickettii* is the most common *Ralstonia* sp. ***R. paucula*** (f. IVc-2) ***R. gilardii*** (*A. faecalis*-like)	No CLSI interpretive criteria. Refer or try Etest value.	Rare in humans as etiologic agent. Probably a nonpathogen. Weak motility. Only MIC can be done and you can only report value, not interpretations. Slow-growing, pinpoint colonies at 24 h on BA.

Respiratory syncytial virus (RSV) An ssRNA negative-sense virus.	For children with mild disease, no specific treatment is necessary other than the treatment of symptoms (e.g., acetaminophen to reduce fever). Children with severe disease may require oxygen therapy and sometimes mechanical ventilation. Ribavirin aerosol may be used in the treatment of some patients with severe disease. Some investigators have used a combination of immune globulin intravenous with high titers of neutralizing RSV antibody and ribavirin to treat patients with compromised immune systems.	RSV is the most common cause of bronchiolitis and pneumonia among infants and children under 1 yr of age. It is spread from person to person. Illness begins most frequently with fever, runny nose, cough, and sometimes wheezing. Most children recover from illness in 8–15 days. The majority of children hospitalized for RSV infection are under 6 mo of age. RSV is a negative-sense, enveloped RNA virus. The virion has an average diameter of between 120 and 300 nm and is unstable in the environment (surviving only a few hours on environmental surfaces), and is readily inactivated with soap and water and disinfectants. Nasopharyngeal wash is a much better diagnostic specimen than a swab. **Serology:** Can request indirect immunofluorescent staining and ELISA to detect antigen.
Rhinosporidium seeberi Not yet cultured in vitro.	No data on therapy.	Causes rhinosporidiosis, a mucosal disease of nasal and other mucosa. This is not a fungus but is a protist from a novel clade of parasites that naturally infect fish and amphibians. Has not yet been cultured and must be diagnosed by direct exam of nasal or other mucosal polyps by observing large round sporangia containing spores.
Rhizomucor The three species in this genus are *R. pusillus, R. miehei, and R. variabilis.*	A combination of surgery and amphotericin B is often used.	A filamentous fungus common in the environment. It can cause serious zygomycosis infections in humans, although rarely. *R. pusillus* and *R. miehei* are thermophilic. Name is derived from its microscopic morphology, which has some similarities with those of both *Rhizopus* and *Mucor.*
Rhizopus The most common isolates are *R. arrhizus, R. azygosporus, R. microsporus, R. schipperae,* and *R. stolonifer.*	Limited therapy data available but treatment is often difficult. Amphotericin B is most often used.	A filamentous fungus, common in nature, that can cause serious and potentially fatal infections in humans. One of the causes of zygomycoses.
Rhodococcus equi Aerobic actinomycete; 12 validly described species.	No CLSI criteria. Use Etest or MIC and report value only. Intracellular location of cells may prevent vancomycin from working, although organism is susceptible in vitro. **1st Rx:** (erythromycin or imipenem) + rifampin, vancomycin **2nd Rx:** ciprofloxacin (variable)	Gram-positive rod (diphtheroid), catalase positive, orange-to-red pigment. Need to rule out *Nocardia* and some *Brevibacterium* spp. with similar pigment.
Rhodotorula Three active species: *R. glutinis, R. minuta,* and *R. mucilaginosa.*	Limited data available, but should be submitted to reference lab for testing. Amphotericin B is most successful.	A yeast found in soil and water; can be opportunistic, mostly in immunocompromised patients. Colonies may be pink, red, orange, or yellow, and cells do not produce pseudohyphae.

Organism	Antimicrobic information	Extent of identification and comments
Rickettsia spp. Small, obligate intracellular bacteria transmitted by arthropods. *R. rickettsii* Causes Rocky Mountain spotted fever; transmitted by tick bites. *R. akari* Causes rickettsialpox, transmitted by mite bites. *R. prowazekii* Causes louse-borne typhus and Brill-Zinsser disease, transmitted via louse feces. *R. typhi* Causes murine typhus, transmitted via flea feces. ***Orientia tsutsugamushi*** Causes scrub typhus, transmitted by chigger bites.	No test method available. **1st Rx:** doxycycline **2nd Rx:** chloramphenicol, fluoroquinolone Relapses can occur after therapy. Call state laboratory for help.	Specimen for diagnosis is blood collected in heparin-containing tube. **Serology:** Latex agglutination, IIF, and Weil-Felix may be requested to confirm diagnosis of RMSF. In the Weil-Felix reaction, *Proteus vulgaris* strain OX-19 reacts strongly with serum from patients with RMSF.
Roseomonas spp. (f. CDC "pink coccoid group") Includes *R. gilardii*, *R. cervicalis*, *R. fauriae*, and three unnamed species.	No CLSI criteria. Refer or try Etest.	Pink, often mucoid; weakly gram-negative, plump, coccoid rods.
Rotavirus	For immunocompetent people, rotavirus gastroenteritis is a self-limited illness. Treatment is nonspecific and consists of oral rehydration therapy to prevent dehydration. About 1 in 40 children with rotavirus gastroenteritis requires hospitalization for intravenous fluids.	Looks like a wheel under electron microscopy (*rota* is Latin for "wheel"). The genome is composed of 11 segments of double-stranded RNA; the virus is stable in the environment. Rotavirus is the most common cause of severe diarrhea among children, resulting in the hospitalization of approximately 55,000 children each year in the United States and the death of over 600,000 children annually worldwide. The incubation period for rotavirus disease is approximately 2 days. The disease is characterized by vomiting and watery diarrhea for 3–8 days, and fever and abdominal pain occur frequently. **Serology:** Secretory IgA is protective. At least five known serotypes. EIA used for antigen detection.
Rothia spp. ***R. dentocariosa*** ***R. mucilaginosa*** (f. *Stomatococcus mucilaginosus*) ***R. nasimurium***	See Diphtheroids. Some *R. dentocariosa* strains have elevated aminoglycoside MICs but good activity with penicillins.	

RSV See Respiratory syncytial virus		
Rubella virus Causes German measles (third disease). An ssRNA virus. Rubella virus is a teratogen, inducing congenital rubella syndrome when spread from mother to fetus in the first trimester of pregnancy.	Live, attenuated vaccine is available.	Rubella was first described by two German physicians in the mid-18th century and recognized as a distinct disease in 1881. It is primarily a respiratory disease that causes a rash and fever for 2–3 days. It is the only togavirus transmitted via the respiratory route. **Serology:** Antibodies appear around the time the rash disappears. Passive hemagglutination, latex agglutination, hemagglutination inhibition, ELISA, and neutralization are available but best used for immune status testing. These tests can detect IgM with rheumatoid factor removed.
Saccharomyces Several species, but *S. cerevisiae* is the most common.	Amphotericin B is the drug of choice for serious infections. The azoles vary in their activity and must be tested by a reference laboratory prior to therapy.	A yeast commonly isolated from human, mammals, birds, wine, beer, fruits, trees, plants, olives, and soil. Also known as "baker's" or "brewer's" yeast. Normally nonpathogenic in competent hosts and may be normal mucosal flora in these individuals.
Salmonella* spp.** ***Salmonella choleraesuis ***Salmonella enteritidis*** ***Salmonella typhi*** *Salmonella enterica* as a representative name was rejected by the Judicial Commission, and *S. choleraesuis* remains the type species; however, a second proposal to reinstate *S. enterica* is before the Commission and a decision should be forthcoming. *S. enterica* is often used in the literature. Responsible for the fourth most common reportable disease in the United States.	K/B, MIC, Etest, but report only ampicillin, fluoroquinolone, and SXT. For *extraintestinal sites*, you can also test and report chloramphenicol and a broad-spectrum cephalosporin. Nalidixic acid can be tested, and if susceptible to fluoroquinolone and resistant to nalidixic acid, then tell doctor the isolate may not be eradicated by fluoroquinolone treatment (21). Ciprofloxacin cannot be used in children younger than 16 yr old. SXT should not be used in newborns (~2 mo) or in women near-term or patients with megaloblastic anemia. Narrow- and expanded-spectrum cephalosporins and aminoglycosides may appear to result in susceptibility in vitro, but do not work in the patient, therefore do not report them (21). Multiple resistances may appear in immigrants. **1st Rx for *S. typhi*:** fluoroquinolone, ceftriaxone (some fluoroquinolone resistance reported) **2nd Rx for *S. typhi*:** chloramphenicol, amoxicillin, or SXT	If a stool isolate has a >95% identification confidence level of *Salmonella* by the system, do a polyvalent and send out results. Send isolate to State. Lysine will always be positive. Confirm the identification of any lysine-negative "*Salmonella*." Most gastroenteritis need not be treated with antibiotics. Therapy for gastrointestinal infection does not shorten illness or decrease time of excretion. Serologically, can request *Salmonella* agglutinins, where a fourfold rise in titer indicates *S. typhi* infection. ELISA detects IgG anti-Vi antibodies to detect carriers.
Scedosporium *S. apiospermum* and *S. prolificans* (f. *S. inflatum*) are the only two species. The sexual state of *S. apiospermum* is *Pseudallescheria boydii*. *S. prolificans* has no sexual stage.	*S. prolificans* is relatively resistant and often refractive to therapy, thus infections can be very serious. Even combination therapies with amphotericin B and azoles are unpredictable. Reference laboratory testing is important. Voriconazole or itraconazole may be considered.	A filamentous, dematiaceous fungus that is opportunistic in humans. *S. prolificans* can infect both competent and immunocompromised patients, usually as arthritis, osteomyelitis, or skin infections.
Schistosoma See Trematodes		

Organism	Antimicrobic information	Extent of identification and comments
Scopulariopsis Several species including a number of anamorphs. The most common species is *S. brevicaulis*, a hyaline mold.	Must be tested for susceptibility. Azoles are not usually helpful in therapy.	Both hyaline and dematiaceous species are in this genus. Usually considered a contaminant but may infect human nails. Many years ago it was associated with death due to metabolizing arsenic in wallpaper to arsine gas, which is highly toxic and smells a little like garlic.
Serratia fonticola	K/B, MIC, Etest. May develop resistance during prolonged therapy with broad-spectrum cephalosporins; therefore retest susceptible isolates within 3–4 days after initiation of therapy (21).	Intrinsic resistance to ampicillin, carbenicillin, and cephalothin (27).
Serratia liquefaciens **group**		
Serratia marcescens Most clinical isolates are not red pigmented, but when they are, they can be nosocomial markers.	Intrinsic resistance to penicillin G, colistin, and cephalothin. May be resistant to ampicillin, carbenicillin, and tetracycline (27). **1st Rx:** broad-spectrum cephalosporin, ertapenem, imipenem, meropenem, or fluoroquinolone **2nd Rx:** aztreonam, gentamicin	
Serratia odorifera		Smells like dirt. Rare in humans.
Serratia plymuthica		Rare in humans.
Serratia rubidea	K/B, MIC, Etest. Use CLSI criteria.	Usually red or orange pigmented. Rare in humans.
Shewanella putrefaciens (f. *Pseudomonas putrefaciens*) Like a glucose-negative *Pseudomonas.*	No CLSI criteria available. MIC only (if desperate).	H_2S positive in triple sugar iron agar butt—unique for a nonfermenter. Ornithine positive—unique for a nonfermenter. Isolated from some wounds. Unknown pathogenicity.
Shigella boydii **(group C)**	K/B, MIC, Etest. Stool AST: report ampicillin, ciprofloxacin, SXT. Nonstool AST: ampicillin, ciprofloxacin, SXT, ceftriaxone (21). For all shigellae: **1st Rx:** fluoroquinolone or azithromycin **2nd Rx:** SXT and ampicillin. Narrow- and expanded-spectrum cephalosporins and aminoglycosides may appear to result in susceptibility in vitro, but don't work well in the patient, so do not report them (21).	Rare in the United States.
Shigella dysenteriae **(group A)**		Rare in the United States.
Shigella flexneri **(group B)**		Often on Native American reservations and in institutions.
Shigella sonnei **(group D)** Shigellae are metabolically inactive *E. coli* organisms, according to *Bergey's*. They belong to the same genetic group. ☣ Shiga toxin is on the select agent list.		Most common in the United States. If identification confidence level of "*Shigella*" is >95%, do group D sera (or send to state lab) and report. Send to state lab. May need to do oxidase test to differentiate *Aeromonas* (oxidase positive) that can cross-react in group D sera. *Shigella* does not invade beyond the lamina propria of intestine. Source is ingestion of contaminated food or water and person-to-person spread. In United States, 450,000 cases/yr with 70 deaths (10).

Simonsiella Belongs to the *Neisseriaceae.*	Refer for testing. One strain tested susceptible to beta-lactams, tetracycline, and gentamicin. Resistant to clindamycin (77).	Normal oral flora. Slight yellow pigment. Fastidious and grows best with serum and yeast extract. Aerobic, gram-negative, crescent-shaped rods often arranged side by side to look like a caterpillar. Exhibits a gliding motility. Grows on blood agar with beta-hemolysis but not on enteric media. *S. muelleri* (humans), *S. crassa* (sheep), *S. steedae* (dogs).

Sinusitis (18)
Viral colds may contribute.
Usually self-limited, lasting 1–3 wk.
Acute: sudden onset. Lasts up to a month.
Subacute: lasts from 4–12 wk.
Chronic: lasts longer than 3 mo.
Recurrent: 4+ episodes within a year, each lasting at least 7 days.

A swab is *not* the specimen of choice, not even from the sinus osteum. Only an aspirate is acceptable.

Organism	Adults (%)	Children (%)
Acute		
S. pneumoniae	34–43	37
H. influenzae	31–35	25
M. catarrhalis	4–5	25
Chronic		
Aerobes	29–43	20 (*Staphylococcus* spp. and *Streptococcus* spp.)
Anaerobes	57–88	80 (*Peptostreptococcus* spp. and *Bacteroides* spp.)

Solobacterium moorei Only one species in genus; rare in humans.	No data available.	Eubacterium-like isolate from human feces (46).
Sphingobacterium multivorum (f. *Flavobacterium* IIk-2) ***Sphingobacterium spiritivorum*** (f. *Flavobacterium* IIk-3)	No CLSI criteria. May have to do Etest or MIC value only.	Nonmotile, catalase positive and oxidase positive, indole negative. Yellow pigment. Rarely associated with serious infections. May appear as rods or coccoid. Nonmotile, catalase positive and oxidase positive, indole negative. Yellow pigment, esculin positive; isolated from blood and urine.
Sphingomonas paucimobilis (f. *Pseudomonas paucimobilis* and IIk-1)		Yellow pigment; oxidase positive; esculin positive; slow growing.
Spirillum minor Causes rat bite fever.	**1st Rx:** amoxicillin-clavulanic acid **2nd Rx:** tetracycline or streptomycin	The Jarisch-Herxheimer reaction (the release of endotoxin when large numbers of organisms are killed by antibiotics) may complicate therapy (66).
Sporothrix *S. schenckii* is the only species. *Ophiostoma stenoceras* is the sexual stage.	Potassium iodide has historically been used as therapy, but amphotericin B, ketoconazole, and itraconazole have also been used.	A thermally dimorphic fungus found normally in the environment but that can cause infections in humans. Sporotrichosis is also called rose handler's disease, since rose thorn pricks of the skin may introduce the fungus, which moves through the lymphatic channels and lymph nodes, producing characteristic lesions along these nodes. Alcoholics may contract pulmonary infection.
Stachybotrys chartarum (f. *S. alternans* and *S. atra*) The only species in this genus.	No susceptibility data available. Refer to reference laboratory.	A filamentous fungus commonly contaminating indoor environments, particularly in water-damaged buildings, where it is associated with "sick-building syndrome." *Stachybotrys* produces trichothecene mycotoxins known as satratoxins that inhibit nucleic acid and protein synthesis.

Organism | **Antimicrobic information** | **Extent of identification and comments**

Organism

Staphylococcus, coagulase negative

S. auricularis

S. capitis

S. cohnii

S. epidermidis
(most common)

S. haemolyticus
(second most common)

S. hominis

S. intermedius
May be slide/tube coagulase positive.

S. lentus

S. lugdunensis
May be slide coagulase positive.

S. sciuri

S. simulans

S. warneri

S. xylosus

Antimicrobic information

K/B, MIC, Etest. Always confirm if resistant to vancomycin or linezolid.
If vancomycin has an MIC of ≥4, confirm it with an Etest or a conventional MIC read at 24 h or brain heart infusion-vancomycin screen plate, or send to reference lab. Do not use disk.
Prolonged therapy with fluoroquinolones can lead to resistance. Initially susceptible isolates may convert after 3–4 days of therapy, and repeat testing may be warranted (21).
Methicillin-resistant isolates should also be reported as resistant to all penicillins, cephems, and other beta-lactams and imipenem because the patient does not respond well to these drugs.
The oxacillin MIC for reporting CoNS as methicillin resistant is ≥0.5.
A disk diffusion test using a 30-μg cefoxitin disk can be used to predict mecA *resistance in CoNS; ≤24 mm is R (21).*
Inducible clindamycin resistance: see "D" test under *S. aureus* below.

S. epidermidis
1st Rx: vancomycin +/− rifampin
2nd Rx: SXT or fluoroquinolone + rifampin

S. haemolyticus
1st Rx: SXT, fluoroquinolone, or nitrofurantoin
2nd Rx: oral cephalosporin

Extent of identification and comments

Between 400 and 700% increase in significant bloodstream infections during the 1980s due to coagulase-negative staphylococci (CoNS) (5).
A single isolate can be significant in a blood culture, so consult the doctor before workup. Use tube coagulase to confirm suspicious latex negatives.
Consider identification to species level if isolate is from a sterile site.

	Bacitracin (0.04 U)	Furazolidone (100 μg)	Lysostaphin (200 μg/ml)	Oxidase
Staphylococcus	R	S	S	–
Micrococcus	S	R	R	+
Stomatococcus	R/S	R/S	R (sticky)	–
Aerococcus	S	S	R	–
Enterococcus	R	S	R	–

Data in table are from reference 6.

Organism

Staphylococcus aureus
Staphylococcus enterotoxins are on the select agent list.

Antimicrobic information

K/B, MIC, Etest. Always confirm if resistant to vancomycin, teicoplanin, linezolid, or quinupristin-dalfopristin.
Keep MRSA and methicillin-susceptible *S. aureus* as two separate and distinct organisms when evaluating AST profiles.
Prolonged therapy with fluoroquinolones can lead to resistance. Initially susceptible isolates may convert after 3–4 days of therapy and repeat testing may be warranted (21).
Methicillin-resistant isolates should also be reported as resistant to all penicillins, cephems, and other beta-lactams and imipenem *because* the patient does not respond well to these drugs (21).
"D" test for clindamycin-inducible resistance: For strains that are resistant to erythromycin and

Extent of identification and comments

A coagulase positive by *any* method is reported as "coagulase positive."
Screen for MRSA with an inhibitory plate or use a cefoxitin 30-μg disk as a *mecA* gene test. Methicillin resistance is chromosomally based, not plasmid based; therefore, a beta-lactamase is not produced. The oxacillin MIC for reporting as MRSA is ≥4 μg/ml.
A disk diffusion test using a 30-μg cefoxitin disk can be used to predict *mecA* resistance: ≤19 mm is R (21). Results are as good as with a probe.
Vancomycin-resistant strains of MRSA are very rare but real. Check anything with a MIC of >4 μg/ml by using a conventional MIC panel or an Etest read after 24 h or a brain heart infusion-vancomycin screen plate, or send to a reference lab. *The disk test is inaccurate in detecting vancomycin-intermediate strains, so do a MIC when zone for vancomycin is ≤14 mm.*
Penicillin-resistant, oxacillin-susceptible strains produce beta-lactamase, and testing a 10-U PEN disk is better than testing an ampicillin disk

<table>
<tr><td></td><td>susceptible to clindamycin. Place 2-μg clindamycin disk 15–26 mm away from a 15-μg erythromycin disk. A flat midzone indicates inducible resistance to clindamycin. This test is not required and should be interpreted with caution in consultation with an infectious disease physician (21).
MRSA
1st Rx: vancomycin
2nd Rx: teicoplanin; SXT
Methicillin-susceptible S. aureus
1st Rx: oxacillin or nafcillin
2nd Rx: narrow-spectrum cephalosporin, vancomycin, or clindamycin</td><td>for K/B testing. For oxacillin-resistant staphylococcus, report as resistant or do not report.
Oxacillin screen plate method: Mueller-Hinton medium + 6 μg of oxacillin/ml + 4% NaCl. Inoculate with swab or spot from 0.5 McFarland standard. Incubate at 35°C for a full 24 h (up to 48 h for CoNS). Any growth = resistance (MRSA) (21).
The screen plate is not a good measure for CoNS resistant to methicillin; use a disk method. When an oxacillin disk is used, the following is necessary (21):
<table><tr><th></th><th>R</th><th>I</th><th>S</th></tr><tr><td>S. aureus</td><td>≤10 mm</td><td>11–12 mm</td><td>≥13 mm</td></tr><tr><td>CoNS</td><td>≤17 mm</td><td></td><td>≥19 mm</td></tr></table></td></tr>
<tr><td>Staphylococcus saprophyticus
Routine testing of urine isolates is not needed, because infections respond to concentrations in urine of common drugs, e.g., SXT, fluoroquinolone, and nitrofurantoin.</td><td></td><td>Although normal on human skin and genitourinary mucosa, causes urinary tract infections in young, sexually active women. Set up a novobiocin disk and look for resistance if urologists actually use the information.</td></tr>
<tr><td>Stenotrophomonas maltophilia
(f. Xanthomonas and Pseudomonas)</td><td>MIC, Etest, (K/B). Use new CLSI guidelines for disk testing of limited drugs.
1st Rx: SXT
2nd Rx: ticarcillin-clavulanate (+/− aztreonam)
Naturally resistant to aminoglycosides and most beta-lactams except ticarcillin-clavulanate (51). Always resistant to carbapenem, imipenem, and ceftriaxone.</td><td>Probably the second most common nonfermenter in the United States. About 85% are susceptible to SXT.
Lysine-positive (rare in nonfermenters) and oxidase-negative nonfermenters. If growing on BA, then is S. maltophilia.</td></tr>
<tr><td>Stomatococcus spp.
Now named Rothia mucilaginosus (6).</td><td>No CLSI guidelines; therefore, resist testing or refer. Try an Etest if necessary.</td><td>Normal human skin, mucosa, and oropharynx flora. Only rare in true infections and not known to be pathogenic. Strongly adherent to agar plate and nonhemolytic.</td></tr>
<tr><td>Streptobacillus moniliformis
SPS is inhibitory.</td><td>No susceptibility test is available for interpretation.
1st Rx: penicillin G active against the bacillus form, but an aminoglycoside or tetracycline must be added to eliminate the L forms
2nd Rx: erythromycin; clindamycin</td><td>Extremely long (100- to 150-μm) filaments can be seen in older cultures. Older cultures may have moniliaceous swellings like a string of pearls that break into coccobacillary forms. This group resembles some mycoplasmas because of its low guanine + cytosine content and it can spontaneously change into L forms (75). Occurs naturally in nasopharynx and oropharynx of wild and lab rats. Human infection is either from rat bites (rat bite fever) or through consumption of contaminated milk or food (Haverhill fever).</td></tr>
<tr><td>Streptococcus, beta-hemolytic
Includes groups A, B, C, G, and F and S. anginosus (“S. milleri”) group (S. constellatus, S. intermedius, and S. anginosus). Most beta-hemolytic streptococci are Voges-Proskauer negative. The “S. milleri” group are small-colony, beta-hemolytic streptococci and are Voges-Proskauer positive.</td><td>Not necessary to test. No penicillin resistance reported in the United States.
If required (after consultation), do K/B, MIC, or Etest per CLSI criteria.
1st Rx: penicillin G or V
2nd Rx: all beta-lactams, erythromycin, azithromycin, clarithromycin</td><td>If isolated from any body site, report it. Do not do susceptibility. If a sterile site, determine grouping. AST only on request.</td></tr>
</table>

Organism	Antimicrobic information	Extent of identification and comments
***Streptococcus*, group G** See *Streptococcus*, beta-hemolytic		
***Streptococcus*, nonhemolytic**	K/B, MIC, Etest.	
Streptococcus*, viridans group** Viridans is not a species name. Species-level identification of viridans blood isolates is to rule out *S. bovis* or other group D streptococci for correlation with colon carcinoma (13). ***S. anginosus ("*S. milleri*" group) ***S. bovis*** ***S. constellatus*** ("*S. milleri*" group) ***S. cristatus*** ***S. hansenii*** ***S. intermedius*** ("*S. milleri*" group) ***S. mitior*** ***S. mitis*** ***S. mutans* group** ***S. oralis*** ***S. parasanguis*** ***S. salivarius* group** ***S. sanguis* group** ***S. sobrinus*** ***S. uberis***	Blood, CSF, bone, and other sterile-site isolates should be tested for penicillin susceptibility by the new CLSI standards. Resistance in this group is emerging in the United States (24). *Most commercial systems are not very good at identifying these isolates.* Do not trust the results if an identification is really important; send it off to a place that knows how to identify them. The "*S. milleri*" group is small-colony, beta-hemolytic group A, C, or G but still considered "viridans group streptococcus," and viridans group interpretive criteria should be used.	Most are vancomycin susceptible, PYR negative, LAP positive, BE negative, NaCl negative. **For sterile sites** **1.** If PYR positive, see *Enterococcus* spp. **2.** If PYR negative, do P-disk to rule out *S. pneumoniae.* **3.** If P-disk is ≥14 mm, see *S. pneumoniae.* **4.** If P-disk is <13 mm but the colony looks like *S. pneumoniae*, repeat P-disk or set up rapid identification method. If the identification confidence is >90%, report it out. If <90% report "*S. viridans*, further identification requires consult." **5.** If P-disk is <13 mm and the colony does not look like *S. pneumoniae*, report "*S. viridans*, no further identification available without consult" (larger institutions may have further test capacity). **For blood isolates** **1.** Rule out *Enterococcus* and *S. pneumoniae.* **2.** If PYR is negative and the P-disk is <13 mm, report "*S. viridans*, susceptibility cannot be done here. Consult lab if needed." (Larger institutions may have additional test capacity.)
***Streptococcus agalactiae* group B**	Not necessary to test. Results are predictable. If required, do MIC or Etest. **1st and 2nd Rx:** same as group A streptococci	PYR negative. **Serology:** Commercial agglutination tests are usually 100% accurate. Rule out beta-hemolytic enterococci with a PYR test. **Spot tests:** Gram-positive cocci, catalase negative, narrow beta-hemolytic with soft periphery on BA, rapid positive (2 h) hippurate or rapid (30 min) CAMP identifies this at 95% (20).

Streptococcus anginosus* group** ***S. anginosus ***S. constellatus*** (beta-hemolytic) ***S. intermedius*** (brain or liver abscess)	Etest if required.	Usually produce a buttery odor.
Streptococcus bovis* group** ***S. alactolyticus ***S. bovis*** Associated with colon cancer. ***S. equinus*** May replace *S. bovis* in nomenclature since it was named first.	Etest if required.	If *S. bovis* isolated from blood, indicate on report the nature of the association with colon cancer. BE positive, NaCl negative, group D positive.
Streptococcus dysgalactiae* subsp. *equisimilis	Etest if required.	Beta-hemolytic.
Streptococcus equi	Etest if required.	Beta-hemolytic, group C streptococcus.
Streptococcus pneumoniae	Penicillin susceptible: **1st Rx:** penicillin **2nd Rx:** multiple agents, e.g., amoxicillin Penicillin resistant (MIC >2.0): **1st Rx:** (i) vancomycin with or without rifampin or (ii) gatifloxacin, levofloxacin, or moxifloxacin **2nd Rx:** For nonmeningeal infections, broad-spectrum and "fourth-generation" cephalosporin, linezolid, antipseudomonal penicillins, or an active fluoroquinolone Naturally resistant to trimethoprim and aminoglycosides. Always confirm if resistant to meropenem, vancomycin, teicoplanin, or linezolid. See beta-hemolytic above.	**Spot tests:** Gram-positive cocci in pairs and chains, catalase negative, alpha-hemolytic on BA with mucoid or flattened colonies, and soluble in 2% or 10% bile identifies this organism at 95% (20). **P-disk procedure** **1.** Streak a quadrant of BA with pure isolate. **2.** Place P-disk on surface. **3.** Incubate overnight, 35°C in 5% CO_2. **4.** Interpretation: ≥14 mm: report as *S. pneumoniae* ≤13 mm: report as viridans group *Streptococcus* **Serology:** Antigen detection by agglutination or electrophoresis is helpful. There are many serotypes. The classic serology test is the quellung, or capsular swelling, test.
Streptococcus pyogenes	No need to do AST on this organism from any site unless the patient is allergic to PEN. Resistance to penicillins, cephalosporins, or vancomycin has *not* been reported in the United States. May need an Etest for erythromycin in penicillin-allergic patients. Erythromycin resistance is low in the United States. **Most beta-hemolytic streptotocci** **1st Rx:** penicillin G or V **2nd Rx:** erythromycin, azithromycin, dirithromycin; clarithromycin; all beta-lactams K/B, MIC, and Etest can be done only if required after consult. For all beta-streptococci, always confirm if resistant to penicillin, vancomycin, teicoplanin, or linezolid.	**Spot test:** Gram-positive cocci in pairs or chains, catalase negative, beta-hemolytic small colonies at 24 h with sharp zone, and a positive PYR identify group A at 95% confidence (20). **Serology:** The beta-hemolytic streptococci were placed into more than 20 serogroups by Rebecca Lancefield. Direct antigen tests are very useful if proper specimens are taken but negatives should still be cultured. Antistreptococcal antibodies appear 2–3 wk after infection with group A. There are about 120 M-protein serotypes. ASO antibodies appear 3–4 weeks after exposure but not in patients with streptococcal skin infections. DNase B and streptozyme may be ordered.

Organism	Antimicrobic information	Extent of identification and comments
Streptomyces Over 3,000 species, with *S. anulatus* (f. *S. griseus*) being the most common, usually as a contaminant. *S. somaliensis* may also be isolated.	No CLSI criteria. Refer. Do not test. Streptomycin in combination with SXT or dapsone has been suggested for treatment.	An aerobic actinomycete. Often a source of antibiotic production. First isolated from patients with mycetomas in what was then French Somaliland. Filamentous bacteria that grow as chalky, somewhat firm colonies in a variety of colors, smell like dirt, and can form aerial filaments. Can cause a white-grain mycetoma.
Suttonella indologenes (f. *Kingella indologenes*) Belongs to the family *Cardiobacteriaceae.*	No CLSI criteria for testing. Susceptibility resembles that of *C. hominis* (45, 75).	Rarely encountered in human flora but may be normal flora (34, 75). Catalase-negative, oxidase-positive, gram-negative rod. Indole positive. Plump, irregularly staining, nonmotile, fastidious organism whose colonies may show spreading or pitting.
Synergistes jonesii Rare in human infection. Newly recognized as colonizers of several body sites.	No data available.	*Synergistes* is a phylotype primarily found in natural environments but recently found in periodontal pockets and caries lesions of humans. Also from peritoneal fluid and soft-tissue infection (42).
Tapeworms ***Diphyllobothrium latum*** **(fish tapeworm)** ***Taenia saginata*** **(beef tapeworm)** ***Taenia solium*** **(pork tapeworm)** ***Dipylidium caninum*** **(dog tapeworm)** ***Hymenolepis nana*** **(dwarf tapeworm)**	**1st Rx:** praziquantel **2nd Rx:** niclosamide	Tapeworms have no alimentary tract, so food must be absorbed through the surface of the worm. All tapeworms of human importance require an intermediate host. *Taenia* sp. eggs have been found in human remains dating back to the Neolithic period, 9000–1500 B.C.
Tatumella ptyseos (f. enteric group 9)	K/B, MIC, Etest.	New member of the *Enterobacteriaceae* isolated from respiratory tract, urine, and blood. "Ptyseos" means "spit." Does not grow very well and is hard to keep on subculture. Unlike other enteric bacteria, this one is motile with a polar or lateral flagellum. Grows best at 25°C. Very rare and opportunistic.
Tetragenococcus **spp.**	No CLSI interpretive criteria. Refer or do Etest.	Gram-positive cocci in clusters and tetrads. No isolates from humans. Old vancomycin-susceptible *Pediococcus* strains placed into this genus. Vancomycin susceptible, PYR negative, LAP positive, BE positive, NaCl positive.

Ticks

Attachment times for disease transmission to humans (4–48 h depending on agent)

Disease	Tick	Attachment time required
Lyme disease (*B. burgdorferi*) (59)	Nymph (*Ixodes dammini*)	36–48 h (10% likely infection)
	Adult (*I. dammini*) (60)	36–48 h
Human granulocytic ehrlichiosis (*Ehrlichia microti*) (69)	Nymph (*I. dammini*)	36 h
Babesiosis (*Babesia microti*) (11)	*I. scapularis* (*I. dammini*)	>24 h
Rickettsia	*Amblyomma* or *Dermacentor*	4–6 h
RMSF (67, 71)	*Dermacentor variabilis*, *D. andersoni*	6–10 h (produces a weak Wasserman test [38])
Relapsing fever (67)	*Ornithodoros* spp.	Not sure (Giemsa smear 70% sensitive for spirochete)

Tinea

A group of dermatophytic fungal diseases also called "ringworm." *Tinea* is the genus name of a moth whose larvae can eat round holes in wool blankets. The red rings seen on the skin of infected individuals apparently looked like these "ringworm" holes in the blankets, hence the name "tinea." These are infections of keratinized tissue (hair, skin, and nails) caused by *Epidermophyton*, *Microsporum*, or *Trichophyton*.

Tinea barbae (ringworm of the beard): *Microsporum* spp. and *Trichophyton* spp.

Tinea capitis (scalp, eyebrows, and lashes): *Microsporum* spp. and *Trichophyton* spp.

Tinea corporis (torso and face): *T. rubrum*, *M. canis*, *T. mentagrophytes*, and others, including *Epidermophyton*

Tinea cruris (jock itch): *T. rubrum*, *E. floccosum*

Tinea nigra (pityriasis nigra): *Hortaea* spp.

Tinea pedis (athlete's foot): *E. floccosum*, *T. mentagrophytes*, *T. rubrum*, and *T. tonsurans*

Tinea unguium (nails): any dermatophyte, yeast, or nondermatophyte mold, *T. rubrum*, *T. mentagrophytes*, and *E. floccosum*

***Toxoplasma* spp.**	**1st Rx:** pyrimethanamine plus sulfadiazine **2nd Rx:** spiramycin	*Toxoplasma* is an obligate intracellular parasite. The intestinal phase occurs in wild and domesticated cats and produces oocysts. The extraintestinal phase may be seen in all infected animals (including cats) and produces tachyzoites and, eventually, bradyzoites or zoitocysts. Toxoplasmosis can be transmitted by ingestion of oocysts (in cat feces) or bradyzoites (in raw or undercooked meat). **Serology:** May request ELISA or IIF for IgG and IgM in acute- and convalescent-phase sera. IgM and IgA used to detect congenital infection.
Trabulsiella guamensis (f. enteric group 90)	K/B, MIC, Etest.	A member of the *Enterobacteraceae* that resembles *Salmonella* but does not agglutinate in *Salmonella* antisera. Rare in humans. Named for L. R. Trabulsi, a Brazilian microbiologist who worked with enteric pathogens. The first isolate was from Guam.

Organism	Antimicrobic information	Extent of identification and comments
Trematodes (flukes; multicellular flatworms) **Causes and sources of infection** Liver flukes: *Fasciola* (from eating watercress), *Clonorchis* (from eating raw fish), *Opisthorchis* (from eating raw fish) Intestinal fluke: *Fasciolopsis* (from eating water chestnuts) Lung fluke: *Paragonimus* (from eating raw crabs or crayfish) Blood fluke: *Schistosoma* (penetrates skin)	**1st Rx:** praziquantel (oral) **For *Fasciola hepatica*** **1st Rx:** triclabendazole	Flukes do not multiply in humans, so the intensity of disease depends on the degree of exposure to infective larvae. Snails are required in the life cycle.
Treponema pallidum	**1st Rx:** penicillins	Noncultivable spirochete that causes syphilis. Observe by dark-field microscopy. Organisms are too thin to be seen on Gram stain. Highly motile with endoflagella. Easily treated, but if untreated, may cause primary, secondary, and late syphilis over a span of many years. **Serology:** Nontreponemal tests: RPR and VDRL. VDRL is the only one approved for CSF testing. Treponemal tests: FTA-ABS and the MHA-TP are most used.
Trichomonas	Metronidazole (90–95% cure rate)	*Trichomonas vaginalis* is a parasite found worldwide. Trichomoniasis is one of the most common sexually transmitted diseases, mainly affecting sexually active women. In North America, it is estimated that more than 8 million new cases are reported yearly.
Trichophyton At least 20 species. The most common are *T. mentagrophytes*, *T. rubrum* (frequently isolated), *T. schoenleinii*, *T. tonsurans*, *T. verrucosum*, and *T. violaceum*. The sexual stage is *Arthroderma*.	The azoles are commonly used for therapy, as are terbinafine, naftifine, and amorolfine.	A dermatophyte that infects hair, skin, and nails. A filamentous fungus.
Trichosporon Genus is undergoing taxonomic revision but *Trichosporon beigelii* (*cutaneum*) is the most significant pathogen among many species in the genus.	Submit to reference laboratory for testing. Amphotericin, fluconazole, and itraconazole are used in treatment of trichosporonosis but MICs are necessary.	A yeast from the environment that can cause potentially serious infections in humans but is also normal flora of mouth, skin, and nails. Causes white piedra, a superficial infection of hair where soft, white nodules are found along the shaft. (Black piedra is caused by *Piedraia hortae.*)
***Trichuris trichiura* (whipworm)** About 60 species of whipworms infect mammals, and *T. trichiura* is the most common human isolate.	Mebendazole or albendazole	The female worm can produce in excess of 10,000 eggs each day, and the worms can live several years in the body.
Tropheryma whipplei Named after George Whipple, who first described Whipple's disease.	No CLSI criteria for testing. **1st Rx:** penicillin G + streptomycin or ceftriaxone for 14 days, then SXT-DS for 1 yr **2nd Rx:** SXT-DS for 14 days, then doxycycline or penicillin VK for 1 yr	Aerobic actinomycete. Cultured and maintained on human embryonic lung fibroblast monolayers but not subcultured on artificial media yet.

***Tsukamurella* spp.** (f. *Gordona* or *Rhodococcus*) Aerobic actinomycetes. Eight species in the genus. *T. inchonensis*, *T. paurometabola*, *T. pulmonis*, *T. strandjordii*, and *T. tyrosinosolvens* have been reported to cause infections in humans.	MIC or Etest or refer. **1st Rx:** erythromycin or rifampin, ciprofloxacin, gentamicin, vancomycin, imipenem	Is diphtheroid-like or a coccobacillus. Cells from colonies are coccobacilli and appear in a zigzag configuration. Nonhemolytic and mucoid. Possibly salmon-pink like *Rhodococcus*. Weakly acid-fast, resistant to lysozyme, urea positive, and nitrate negative. (Similar to *Gordona* spp.). Has mycolic acid in the cell walls. Can be an opportunist in humans. The first human isolate of *Tsukamurella* was reported in 1971 as *Gordona aurantiaca* and was from the sputum of a TB patient. The type strain *T. paurometabola* was first isolated from the ovaries of bedbugs.
Turicella otitidis The only species in its genus.	If from tympanocentesis, report MIC value only, no interpretation. Most MICs are low, but this species can be resistant to macrolides and clindamycin (36).	Would likely be reported as "diphtheroid." Catalase positive, nonmotile, oxidizer. Commonly isolated from ears but does not cause otitis media with effusion in children. Strongly CAMP positive.
Ureaplasma urealyticum	No test done. **1st Rx:** doxycycline **2nd Rx:** erythromycin (best for pregnant women)	Commonly found in the urogenital tract of sexually active adolescents and adults. Microscopy and serology not useful. No commercial tests available. PCR amplification available but less useful than culture. Organisms very labile. Must use appropriate transport. Recover organisms on Shepard's 10B urea broth and 8A urea agar. Culture positive in 1–2 days.
***Ustilago* spp.** Rare cause of disease in humans.	No data available.	A member of the smut fungi; an environmental organism whose spores can be cultured in vitro to grow as a yeast (basidiospores). May cause type I allergies like hay fever and asthma.
***Vagococcus* spp.**	No CLSI interpretive criteria. Refer or do Etest.	Gram-positive cocci in chains. Vancomycin susceptible, PYR positive, LAP positive, BE positive, NaCl positive. *Vagococcus* resembles *Enterococcus*, but *V. fluvialis*, the species usually found in human infections, is motile. The motile enterococci (*E. gallinarum* and *E. casseliflavus*) should have elevated vancomycin MICs (*vanC* gene) and are vancomycin intermediate and nonmotile, while *Vagococcus* is vancomycin susceptible and motile.
Varicella-zoster virus (VZV) Varicella = chicken pox. Zoster = shingles. Testing for varicella-zoster is part of the diagnostic algorithm to rule out smallpox diagnosis.	An effective vaccine is available. Varicella-zoster immune globulin may be helpful but is short-lived. Acyclovir is recommended for persons who are more likely to develop serious chicken pox and must be given within 24 h of the appearance of symptoms.	Chicken pox occurs mostly in children <15 yr old. The rash appears first on the trunk and face, but can spread over the entire body causing 250 to 500 itchy blisters. Shingles, or herpes zoster, is caused by the chicken pox virus that remains in the nerve roots of all persons who have had chicken pox and can emerge years later to cause a painful illness. Persons who have not had chicken pox can be infected by a patient suffering from shingles. One cannot "catch" shingles from another shingles-infected person. **Serology:** IIF and passive hemagglutination (for immune status), ELISA, CF. IgM and IgG antibodies to VZV found in patients with shingles.
Vibrio alginolyticus	No CLSI interpretive criteria. **1st Rx:** doxycycline + ceftazidime **2nd Rx:** cefotaxime or fluoroquinolone	Opportunist in wounds; does not usually cause gastrointestinal disease.

Organism	Antimicrobic information	Extent of identification and comments
Vibrio cholerae Only serotype O1 causes cholera. El Tor is hardier, survives longer in environment, grows best in the lab, and is more resistant to drugs. Classical: not as dangerous.	CLSI interpretive criteria are available for *V. cholerae* only if the special method is used (21). MIC and K/B can be used for ampicillin, tetracycline, SXT, and sulfonamides. K/B cannot be used for erythromycin because of poor correlation with MIC results (21). ***V. cholerae*** **1st Rx:** doxycycline or fluoroquinolone **2nd Rx:** SXT (strain O139 is resistant to SXT) For other vibrios, MIC values or Etest values can be reported but not S-I-R. *Fluid replacement therapy is critical.*	Infectious dose is 10^8 organisms/ml. Lumen of small intestine is where exotoxin is bound and absorbed by ganglioside of intestinal epithelial cells. Increased cAMP and decreased Na absorption; increased Cl excretion. **Serology:** A coagglutination assay detects *V. cholerae* antigens in stool. A vibriocidal assay detects IgM antibodies.
Vibrio damsela (f. EF-5)	***V. damsela*** **1st Rx:** doxycycline + ceftazidime **2nd Rx:** cefotaxime or fluoroquinolone	Causes lesions in damselfish. One-half of cultures come from fish or marine animals, one-half from human wounds.
Vibrio fluvialis (f. EF-6) Causes sporadic diarrhea (49).		Requires NaCl in all media. GI illness is due to presence in seawater or oysters.
Vibrio furnissii (f. EF-6) May be same as *V. fluvialis.*		
Vibrio hollisae (f. EF-13) Causes sporadic diarrhea.		GI disease and diarrhea. NaCl required for growth in all media. May be in pure culture from stool of infected patients.
Vibrio mimicus Mimics *V. cholerae* non-O1.		
Vibrio parahaemolyticus Causes gastroenteritis with an incubation period of ~15 h. Mostly from seafood.	Supportive therapy. **1st Rx:** antibiotic therapy does not decrease course. Sensitive to fluoroquinolone and doxycycline.	
Vibrio vulnificus (f. *Beneckea vulnifica*) Mostly causes septicemia (days after eating raw oysters) and wound infections (associated with sea water)	No CLSI criteria for testing. Refer. **1st Rx:** doxycycline + ceftazidime **2nd Rx:** cefotaxime or fluoroquinolone	Requires NaCl for growth. Lysine and ornithine positive. Sometimes called "lactose-positive *Vibrio.*" Associated with septicemia and local lesions.
VZV See Varicella-zoster virus		

Wangiella dermatitidis The only species in its genus. Some experts still use *Exophiala dermatitidis* as the correct name; see above.	Optimal treatment not well documented. Amphotericin B alone or in combination with ketoconazole and rifampin has been used.	A dematiaceous fungus that is common in nature and can cause infection in humans.
Weeksella virosa (f. IIf)	No CLSI interpretive criteria. Refer.	Gram-negative, slightly pleomorphic rods. Cells sometimes appear thin in the center with thickened ends, the so-called II-forms. Nonmotile, MacConkey negative, oxidase positive, weak indole positive. Mucoid and sticky; hard to remove from agar. Mostly from female urinary tract. Grows on Thayer-Martin agar.
Weeksella zoohelcum (f. IIj; new name: *Bergeyella zoohelcum*)		Gram-negative, medium to long rod. Oxidase positive, MacConkey negative, indole and urea positive. Seen in human wounds, often from animal bites or scratches. Colonies may adhere to plate (especially with rabbit BA).
West Nile virus	No specific therapy available.	In 2005, 2,950 cases were reported in the United States. A neurotropic arbovirus carried by mosquitoes. Natural host is likely migrating or local birds. Disease may vary from mild to life threatening.
Whipple's disease See *Tropheryma whipplei*		
Xenorhabdus	Do not test.	New member of the *Enterobacteriaceae* found only in nematodes.
Yersinia enterocolitica	K/B, MIC, Etest. **1st Rx:** SXT or fluoroquinolone **2nd Rx:** broad-spectrum cephalosporin or antipseudomonal aminoglycoside	U.S. strains are usually indole positive; European strains are usually indole negative. Use cefsulodin-Irgasan-novobiocin agar if *Y. enterocolitica* is requested, and report out at 72 h. Environmental, diarrhea, septicemia, mesenteric lymphadenitis, blood product contaminant.
Yersinia frederiksenii Formerly in the *Y. enterocolitica* group.		Environmental, rare in humans.
Yersinia intermedia Formerly in the *Y. enterocolitica* group.		Environmental, rare in humans.
Yersinia kristensenii	K/B, MIC, Etest.	Environmental, rare in humans.
Yersinia pestis ☣	Refer for safety reasons. Ensure testing for gentamicin, streptomycin, tetracycline, ciprofloxacin, chloramphenicol, and SXT. *Do not test or report beta-lactams; they do not work (21).* **1st Rx:** streptomycin; gentamicin or tobramycin **2nd Rx:** chloramphenicol or doxycycline; also susceptible to fluoroquinolone and SXT in vitro	See bipolar stain with Gram, Giemsa, and Wright's stains. Bipolarity may be lost on subculture. Also, *Y. pestis* grows as clumps at the bottom and sides of broth tube, while *Y. pseudotuberculosis* grows as a smooth suspension in the broth.

Organism	Antimicrobic information	Extent of identification and comments
Yersinia pseudotuberculosis	K/B, MIC, Etest.	Mesenteric lymphadenitis, diarrhea, septicemia.
Yersinia ruckeri		Causes a disease in trout; rare in humans.
Yokenella regensburgei (f. enteric group 45)	K/B, MIC, Etest.	New member of the *Enterobacteriaceae* isolated from feces, wounds, respiratory system, knee joints.
Zygomycetes	This is a class of fungi with fluffy, cottony growth in the laboratory that produce broad hyphae and exhibit spores in a saclike structure called a sporangium. Most are opportunistic pathogens, but they can occasionally cause severe disease, mostly in immunocompromised patients. Two orders are represented in the *Zygomycetes*: the *Mucorales* and the *Entomophthorales*, which are less common.	

References

1. **Abbott, S. L.** 2003. *Klebsiella, Enterobacter, Citrobacter, Serratia, Plesiomonas*, and other *Enterobacteriaceae*, p. 684–700. *In* P. R. Murray, E. J. Baron, J. H. Jorgensen, M. A. Pfaller, and R. H. Yolken (ed.), *Manual of Clinical Microbiology*, 8th ed. ASM Press, Washington, DC.

2. **American Academy of Pediatrics.** 2003. *Red Book*. American Academy of Pediatrics, Elk Grove Village, IL.

3. **Anzai, Y., Y. Kudo, and H. Oyaizu.** 1997. The phylogeny of the genera *Chryseomonas, Flavimonas*, and *Pseudomonas* supports synonymy of these three genera. *Int. J. Syst. Bacteriol.* **47**:249–251.

4. **Banck, G., and M. Nyman.** 1986. Tonsillitis and rash associated with *Corynebacterium haemolyticum*. *J. Infect. Dis.* **154**:1037–1040.

5. **Banerjee, S. N., T. G. Emori, D. H. Culver, R. P. Gaynes, W. R. Jarvis, T. Horan, J. R. Edwards, J. Tolson, T. Henderson, W. J. Martone, and the National Nosocomial Infections Surveillance System.** 1991. Secular trends in nosocomial primary bloodstream infections in the United States, 1980–1989. *Am. J. Med.* **91**(Suppl. 3B):86–89.

6. **Bannerman, T. L.** 2003. *Staphylococcus, Micrococcus*, and other catalase-positive cocci that grow aerobically, p. 384–404. *In* P. R. Murray, E. J. Baron, J. H. Jorgensen, M. A. Pfaller, and R. H. Yolken (ed.), *Manual of Clinical Microbiology*, 8th ed. ASM Press, Washington, DC.

7. **Barenfanger, J.** 1990. Identification of yeasts and other fungi from direct microscopic examination of clinical specimens. *Clin. Microbiol. Newsl.* **12**:9–16.

8. **Baron, E. J., M. P. Weinstein, W. M. Dunne, Jr., P. Yagupsky, D. F. Welch, and D. M. Wilson.** 2005. *Cumitech 1C, Blood Cultures IV.* Coordinating ed., E. J. Baron. ASM Press, Washington, DC.

9. **Black, J. A., E. S. Moland, and K. S. Thomson.** 2005. AmpC disk test for detection of plasmid-mediated *ampC* β-lactamases in *Enterobacteriaceae* lacking chromosomal *ampC* β-lactamases. *J. Clin. Microbiol.* **43**:3110–3113.

10. **Bopp, C. A., F. W. Brenner, P. I. Fields, J. G. Wells, and N. A. Strockbine.** 2003. *Escherichia, Shigella*, and *Salmonella*, p. 654–671. *In* P. R. Murray, E. J. Baron, J. H. Jorgensen, M. A. Pfaller, and R. H. Yolken (ed.), *Manual of Clinical Microbiology*, 8th ed. ASM Press, Washington, DC.

11. **Boustani, M. R., and J. A. Gelfand.** 1996. Babesiosis. *Clin. Infect. Dis.* **22:**611–615.

12. **Brouqui, P., T. J. Marrie, and D. Raoult.** 2003. *Coxiella*, p. 1030–1036. *In* P. R. Murray, E. J. Baron, J. H. Jorgensen, M. A. Pfaller, and R. H. Yolken (ed.), *Manual of Clinical Microbiology*, 8th ed. ASM Press, Washington, DC.

13. **Bryan, C. S.** 1989. Clinical implications of positive blood cultures. *Clin. Microbiol. Rev.* **2:**329–353.

14. **Carlson, P., S. Kontiainen, and O. V. Renkonen.** 1994. Antimicrobial susceptibility of *Arcanobacterium haemolyticum*. *Antimicrob. Agents Chemother.* **38:**142–143.

15. **Centers for Disease Control and Prevention.** 1991. Epidemiologic notes and reports. Foodborne outbreak of gastroenteritis caused by *Escherichia coli* O157:H7—North Dakota, 1990. *Morb. Mortal. Wkly. Rep.* **40:**265–267.

16. **Centers for Disease Control and Prevention.** 1997. Gonorrhea among men who have sex with men—selected sexually transmitted disease clinics, 1993–1996. *Morb. Mortal. Wkly. Rep.* **46:**889–892.

17. **Chin-Hong, P. V., D. A. Sutton, M. Roemer, M. A. Jacobson, and J. A. Aberg.** 2001. Invasive fungal sinusitis and meningitis due to *Arthrographis kalrae* in a patient with AIDS. *J. Clin. Microbiol.* **39:**804–807.

18. **Chow, A. W.** 2004. Infections of the sinuses and parameningeal structures, p. 428–443. *In* S. L. Gorbach, J. G. Bartlett, and N. R. Blacklow (ed.), *Infectious Diseases*, 3rd ed. Lippincott Williams & Wilkins, Philadelphia, PA.

19. **Clarridge, J. E.** 1989. The recognition and significance of *Arcanobacterium haemolyticum*. *Clin. Microbiol. Newsl.* **11:**41–48.

20. **Clinical and Laboratory Standards Institute.** 2002. *Abbreviated Identification of Bacteria and Yeast.* Standard M35-A. CLSI, Wayne, PA.

21. **Clinical and Laboratory Standards Institute.** 2006. *Performance Standards for Antimicrobial Susceptibility Testing: Sixteenth Informational Supplement.* CLSI, Wayne, PA.

22. **Coyle, M. B., and B. A. Lipsky.** 1990. Coryneform bacteria in infectious diseases: clinical and laboratory aspects. *Clin. Microbiol. Rev.* **3:**227–246.

23. **Doctor Fungus.** www.doctorfungus.com.

24. **Doern, G. V., M. J. Ferraro, A. B. Brueggeman, K. L. Ruoff.** 1996. Emergence of high rates of antimicrobial resistance among viridans group streptococci in the United States, 1993–1996. *Antimicrob. Agents Chemother.* **40:**891–894.

25. **Dunne, W. M., Jr., and D. J. Hardin.** 2005. Use of several inducer and substrate antibiotic combinations in a disk approximation assay format to screen for *ampC* induction in patient isolates of *Pseudomonas aeruginosa*, *Enterobacter* spp., *Citrobacter* spp., and *Serratia* spp. *J. Clin. Microbiol.* **43:**5945–5949.

26. **Emancipator, K.** 1997. Critical values: ASCP practice parameter. *Am. J. Clin. Pathol.* **108:**247–253.

27. **Farmer, J. J.** 2003. *Enterobacteriaceae*: introduction and identification, p. 636–653. *In* P. R. Murray, E. J. Baron, J. H. Jorgensen, M. A. Pfaller, and R. H. Yolken (ed.), *Manual of Clinical Microbiology*, 8th ed. ASM Press, Washington, DC.

28. **Farmer, J. J., III, J. M. Janda, and K. Birkhead.** 2003. *Vibrio*, p. 706–718. *In* P. R. Murray, E. J. Baron, J. H. Jorgensen, M. A. Pfaller, and R. H. Yolken (ed.), *Manual of Clinical Microbiology*, 8th ed. ASM Press, Washington, DC.

29. **Folds, J. D., and D. E. Normansell.** 1999. *Pocket Guide to Clinical Immunology.* ASM Press, Washington, DC.

30. **Forbes, B. A., D. F. Sahm, and A. S. Weissfeld.** 1998. *Bailey and Scott's Diagnostic Microbiology*, 10th ed., p. 586–589. Mosby, St. Louis, MO.

31. **Forbes, B. A., D. F. Sahm, and A. S. Weissfeld.** 1998. *Bailey and Scott's Diagnostic Microbiology*, 10th ed., p. 340–349. Mosby, St. Louis, MO.

32. **Forbes, B. A., D. F. Sahm, and A. S. Weissfeld.** 1998. *Bailey and Scott's Diagnostic Microbiology*, 10th ed., p. 305–320. Mosby, St. Louis, MO.

33. **Forbes, B. A., D. F. Sahm, and A. S. Weissfeld.** 1998. *Bailey and Scott's Diagnostic Microbiology*, 10th ed., p. 673–685. Mosby, St. Louis, MO.

34. **Forbes, B. A., D. F. Sahm, and A. S. Weissfeld.** 1998. *Bailey and Scott's Diagnostic Microbiology*, 10th ed., p. 541–546. Mosby, St. Louis, MO.

35. **Forbes, B. A., D. F. Sahm, and A. S. Weissfeld.** 1998. *Bailey and Scott's Diagnostic Microbiology*, 10th ed., p. 488–500. Mosby, St. Louis, MO.

36. **Funke, G., and K. A. Bernard.** 2003. Coryneform gram-positive rods, p. 472–501. *In* P. R. Murray, E. J. Baron, J. H. Jorgensen, M. A. Pfaller, and R. H. Yolken (ed.), *Manual of Clinical Microbiology*, 8th ed. ASM Press, Washington, DC.

37. **Garcia, L. S., and D. A. Bruckner.** 1993. *Diagnostic Medical Parasitology*, 2nd ed. ASM Press, Washington, DC.

38. **Garin, C., and A. Bujadoux.** 1993. Paralysis by ticks. *Clin. Infect. Dis.* **16:**168–169.

39. **Gilbert, D. N., R. D. Moellering, Jr., G. M. Eliopoulos, and M. A. Sande.** 2005. *The Sanford Guide to Antimicrobial Therapy*, 35th ed. Antimicrobial Therapy, Inc., Hyde Park, VT.

40. **Gilligan, P. H., G. Lum, P. A. R. Vandamme, and S. Whittier.** 2003. *Burkholderia, Stenotrophomonas, Ralstonia, Brevundimonas, Comamonas, Delftia, Pandoraea*, and *Acidovorax*, p. 729–748. *In* P. R. Murray, E. J. Baron, J. H. Jorgensen, M. A. Pfaller, and R. H. Yolken (ed.), *Manual of Clinical Microbiology*, 8th ed. ASM Press, Washington, DC.

41. **Hall, M., L. Hoyt, P. Ferrieri, P. M. Schlievert, and H. B. Jenson.** 1999. Kawasaki syndrome-like illness associated with infection caused by enterotoxin B-secreting *Staphylococcus aureus. Clin. Infect. Dis.* **29:**586–589.

41a. **Helsel, L. O., D. Hollis, A. G. Steigerwalt, R. E. Morey, J. Jordan, T. Aye, J. Radosevic, D. Jannat-Khah, D. Thiry, D. R. Lonsway, J. B. Patel, M. I. Daneshvar, and P. N. Levett.** 2007. Identification of "*Haematobacter*," a new genus of aerobic gram-negative rods isolated from clinical specimens, and reclassification of *Rhodobacter massiliensis* as "*Haematobacter massiliensis* comb. nov." *J. Clin. Microbiol.* **45:**1238–1243.

42. **Horz, H.-P., D. M. Citron, Y. A. Warren, E. J. C. Goldstein, and G. Conrads.** 2006. *Synergistes* group organisms of human origin. *J. Clin. Microbiol.* **44:**2914–2920.

43. **Howanitz, P. J., S. J. Steindel, and N. V. Heard.** 2002. Laboratory critical values policies and procedures. A College of American Pathologists Q-Probes study in 623 institutions. *Arch. Pathol. Lab. Med.* **126:**663–669.

44. **Isenberg, H. D. (ed.).** 2004. *Clinical Microbiology Procedures Handbook*, 2nd ed. ASM Press, Washington, DC.

45. **Jenny, D. B., P. W. Letendre, and G. Iverson.** 1987. Endocarditis caused by *Kingella indologenes. Rev. Infect. Dis.* **9:**787–789.

45a. **Jorgensen, J. H., and M. A. Pfaller.** 2004. *A Clinician's Dictionary of Pathogenic Microorganisms.* ASM Press, Washington, DC.

46. **Kageyama, A., and Y. Benno.** 2000. Phylogenetic and phenotypic characterization of some *Eubacterium*-like isolates from human feces: description of *Solobacterium moorei* gen. nov., sp. nov. *Microbiol. Immunol.* **44:**223–227.

47. **Kost, G. J.** 1990. Critical limits for urgent clinician notification at US medical centers. *JAMA* **263:**704–707.

48. **Larone, D. H.** 2002. *Medically Important Fungi. A Guide to Identification*, 4th ed. ASM Press, Washington, DC.

49. **Lee, J. V., P. Shread, A. L. Furniss, and T. N. Bryant.** 1981. Taxonomy and description of *Vibrio fluvialis* sp. nov. (synonym group F vibrios, group EF-6). *J. Appl. Bacteriol.* **50:**73–94.

50. **Levett, P. N.** 2003. *Leptospira* and *Leptonema*, p. 929–936. *In* P. R. Murray, E. J. Baron, J. H. Jorgensen, M. A. Pfaller, and R. H. Yolken (ed.), *Manual of Clinical Microbiology*, 8th ed. ASM Press, Washington, DC.

51. **Livermore, D. M., T. G. Winstanley, and K. P. Shannon.** 2001. Interpretative reading: recognizing the unusual and inferring resistance mechanisms from resistance phenotypes. *J. Antimicrob. Chemother.* **48**(Suppl. S1)**:**87–102.

52. **Logan, N. S., and P. C. B. Turnbull.** 2003. *Bacillus* and other aerobic endospore-forming bacteria, p. 445–460. *In* P. R. Murray, E. J. Baron, J. H. Jorgensen, M. A. Pfaller, and R. H. Yolken (ed.), *Manual of Clinical Microbiology*, 8th ed. ASM Press, Washington, DC.

53. **Mahony, J. B., B. K. Coombes, and M. A. Chernesky.** 2003. *Chlamydia* and *Chlamydophila*, p. 991–1004. *In* P. R. Murray, E. J. Baron, J. H. Jorgensen, M. A. Pfaller, and R. H. Yolken (ed.), *Manual of Clinical Microbiology*, 8th ed. ASM Press, Washington, DC.

54. **Mason, W. H., and M. Takahashi.** 1999. Kawasaki syndrome. *Clin. Infect. Dis.* **28:**169–185.

54a. **Mathisen, G. P., and J. P. Johnson.** 1997. Brain abscess. *Clin. Infect. Dis.* **25:**763–779.

55. **Medical Letter, Inc.** 1997. Treatment of Lyme disease. *Med. Lett. Drugs Ther.* **39:**47–48.

56. **Montejo, J. M., I. Alberola, P. Glez-Zarate, A. Alvarez, J. Alonso, A. Canovas, and C. Aguirre.** 1993. Open, randomized therapeutic trial of six antimicrobial regimens in the treatment of human brucellosis. *Clin. Infect. Dis.* **16:**671–676.

57. **Nachamkin, I.** 2003. *Campylobacter* and *Arcobacter*, p. 902–914. *In* P. R. Murray, E. J. Baron, J. H. Jorgensen, M. A. Pfaller, and R. H. Yolken (ed.), *Manual of Clinical Microbiology*, 8th ed. ASM Press, Washington, DC.

58. **Nolte, F. S., K. E. Arnold, H. Sweat, E. F. Winton, and G. Funke.** 1996. Vancomycin-resistant *Aureobacterium* species cellulitis and bacteremia in a patient with acute myelogenous leukemia. *J. Clin. Microbiol.* **34:**1992–1994.

59. **Piesman, J.** 1993. Dynamics of *Borrelia burgdorferi* transmission by nymphal *Ixodes dammini* ticks. *J. Infect. Dis.* **167:**1082–1085.

60. **Piesman, J., G. O. Maupin, E. G. Campos, and C. M. Happ.** 1991. Duration of adult *Ixodes dammini* attachment and transmission of *Borrelia burgdorferi*, with description of a needle aspiration isolation method. *J. Infect. Dis.* **163:**895–897.

61. **Reimer, L. G., M. L. Wilson, and M. P. Weinstein.** 1997. Update on detection of bacteremia and fungemia. *Clin. Microbiol. Rev.* **10:**444–465.

62. **Riegel, P., D. de Briel, G. Prévost, F. Jehl, and H. Monteil.** 1994. Genomic diversity among *Corynebacterium jeikeium* strains and comparison with biochemical characteristics and antimicrobial susceptibilities. *J. Clin. Microbiol.* **32:**1860–1865.

63. **Ruoff, K. L.** 2003. *Aerococcus, Abiotrophia,* and other infrequently isolated aerobic catalase-negative, gram-positive cocci, p. 434–444. *In* P. R. Murray, E. J. Baron, J. H. Jorgensen, M. A. Pfaller, and R. H. Yolken (ed.), *Manual of Clinical Microbiology*, 8th ed. ASM Press, Washington, DC.

63a. **Schreckenberger, P. C., M. I. Daneshvar, and D. G. Hollis.** 2007. *Acinetobacter, Achromobacter, Chryseobacterium, Moraxella,* and other nonfermentative gram-negative rods, p. 770–802. *In* P. R. Murray, E. J. Baron, J. H. Jorgensen, M. L. Landry, and M. A. Pfaller (ed.), *Manual of Clinical Microbiology,* 9th ed. ASM Press, Washington, DC.

64. **Shapiro, E. D., M. A. Gerber, N. B. Holabird, A. T. Berg, H. M. Feder, Jr., G. L. Bell, P. N. Rys, and D. H. Persing.** 1992. A controlled trial of antimicrobial prophylaxis for Lyme disease after deer tick bites. *N. Engl. J. Med.* **327:**1769–1773.

65. **Soriano, F., J. M. Aguado, C. Ponte, R. Fernandez-Roblez, and J. L. Rodriquez-Tudela.** 1990. Urinary tract infection caused by *Corynebacterium* D2: report of 82 cases and review. *Rev. Infect. Dis.* **12:**1019–1034.

66. **Spach, D. H., and W. C. Liles.** 1999. Antimicrobial therapy for bacterial diseases, p. 337–348. *In* R. K. Root, F. Waldvogel, L. Corey, and W. E. Stamm (ed.), *Clinical Infectious Diseases: A Practical Approach.* Oxford University Press, New York, NY.

67. **Spach, D. H., W. C. Liles, G. L. Campbell, R. E. Quick, D. E. Anderson, Jr., and T. R. Fritsche.** 1993. Tick-borne diseases in the United States. *N. Engl. J. Med.* **329:**936–947.

68. **Stout, J. E., J. D. Rihs, and V. L. Yu.** 2003. *Legionella,* p. 809–823. *In* P. R. Murray, E. J. Baron, J. H. Jorgensen, M. A. Pfaller, and R. H. Yolken (ed.), *Manual of Clinical Microbiology*, 8th ed. ASM Press, Washington, DC.

69. **Telford, S. R., III.** 1997. Risk for acquiring human granulocytic ehrlichiosis: exposure to deer blood or deer ticks? *Clin. Infect. Dis.* **24:**531–533.

70. **Thomson, R. B., and J. M. Miller.** 2003. Specimen collection, transport, and processing: bacteriology, p. 286–330. *In* P. R. Murray, E. J. Baron, J. H. Jorgensen, M. A. Pfaller, and R. H. Yolken (ed.), *Manual of Clinical Microbiology*, 8th ed. ASM Press, Washington, DC.

71. **Thorner, A. R., D. H. Walker, and W. A. Petri, Jr.** 1998. Rocky mountain spotted fever. *Clin. Infect. Dis.* **27:**1353–1359.

72. **Tuohy, M. J., G. W. Procop, and J. A. Washington.** 2000. Antimicrobial susceptibility of *Abiotrophia adiacens* and *Abiotrophia defectiva. Diagn. Microbiol. Infect. Dis.* **38:** 189–191.

73. **Tuuminen, T., T. Heinäsmäki, and T. Kerttula.** 2006. First report of bacteremia by *Asaia bogorensis*, in a patient with a history of intravenous-drug abuse. *J. Clin. Microbiol.* **44:**3048–3050.

74. **Vogel, B. F., K. Venkateswaran, H. Christensen, E. Falsen, G. Christiansen, and L. Gram.** 2000. Polyphasic taxonomic approach in the description of *Alishewanella fetalis* gen. nov., sp. nov., isolated from a human foetus. *Int. J. Syst. Evol. Microbiol.* **50:**1133–1142.

75. **von Graevenitz, A., R. Zbinden, and R. Mutters.** 2003. *Actinobacillus, Capnocytophaga, Eikenella, Kingella, Pasteurella,* and other fastidious or rarely encountered

gram-negative rods, p. 609–622. *In* P. R. Murray, E. J. Baron, J. H. Jorgensen, M. A. Pfaller, and R. H. Yolken (ed.), *Manual of Clinical Microbiology*, 8th ed. ASM Press, Washington, DC.

76. **Welch, D. F., and L. N. Slater.** 2003. *Bartonella* and *Afipia*, p. 824–834. *In* P. R. Murray, E. J. Baron, J. H. Jorgensen, M. A. Pfaller, and R. H. Yolken (ed.), *Manual of Clinical Microbiology*, 8th ed. ASM Press, Washington, DC.

77. **Whitehouse, R. L., H. Jackson, M. C. Jackson, and M. M. Ramji.** 1987. Isolation of *Simmonsiella* sp. from a neonate. *J. Clin. Microbiol.* **25:**522–525.

78. **Xi, L., K. Fukushima, C. Lu, K. Takizawa, R. Liao, and K. Nishimura.** 2004. First case of *Arthrographis kalrae* ethmoid sinusitis and ophthalmitis in the People's Republic of China. *J. Clin. Microbiol.* **42:**4828–4831.

79. **Yamada, Y., K. Katsura, H. Kawasaki, Y. Widyastuti, S. Saono, T. Seki, T. Uchimura, and K. Komagata.** 2000. *Asaia bogorensis* gen. nov., sp. nov., an unusual acetic acid bacterium in the α-*Proteobacteria*. *Int. J. Syst. Evol. Microbiol.* **50:**823–829.

Index

A

B

C

D

E

F

G

H

I

U

V

W

X

Y

Z